编辑委员会

患者自杀风险管理指导手册
（汉英对照）

Guidance Manual for Suicide Risk Management of Patients

（Bilingual in English and Chinese）

主　编◎胡德英　刘义兰　孙　晖
主　审◎童永胜　郭　鑫

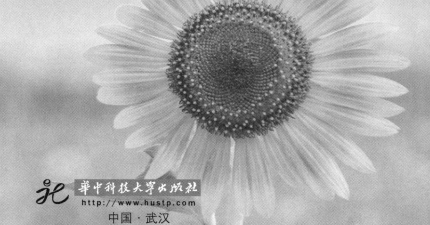

华中科技大学出版社
http://www.hustp.com
中国·武汉

图书在版编目（CIP）数据

患者自杀风险管理指导手册：汉英对照 / 胡德英，刘义兰，孙晖主编 . — 武汉 ：华中科技大学出版社，2020.12
ISBN 978-7-5680-6732-4

Ⅰ . ①患… Ⅱ . ①胡… ②刘… ③孙… Ⅲ . ①病人-自杀-风险管理-手册-汉、英 Ⅳ . ①R197.323.2-62

中国版本图书馆CIP数据核字（2020）第239969号

患者自杀风险管理指导手册（汉英对照）　　　　　　　　　　　　　　胡德英 刘义兰 孙晖
Huanzhe Zisha Fengxian Guanli Zhidao Shouce（Hanying Duizhao）　　　　　　　主编

策划编辑：刘　平　荣　静
责任编辑：刘　平
封面设计：原色设计
责任校对：封力煊
责任监印：周治超
出版发行：华中科技大学出版社（中国•武汉）　　　电话：(027)81321913
　　　　　武汉市东湖新技术开发区华工科技园　　　邮编：430223
录　　排：湖北新华印务有限公司
印　　刷：武汉科源印刷设计有限公司
开　　本：710mm×1000mm　1/16
印　　张：13.5
字　　数：255千字
版　　次：2020年12月第1版第1次印刷
定　　价：48.00元

序

　　自杀是一个非常严重的公共卫生问题。根据世界卫生组织（WHO）发表的全球自杀报告，每年有80多万人死于自杀，在我国，每10万人中有9.7人自杀。医院管理以患者为中心，以质量安全为核心，预防患者自杀不良事件发生，保障患者安全是医院的重要职责与任务。

　　当前中国正处于社会转型期的特殊情境之下，与之伴随的社会心理问题日益突出，患者自杀问题尚未引起足够重视。"住院患者自杀身亡，医患双方对簿公堂"的案例时有发生。患者自杀给家属、同室病友、值班医务人员等带来强烈的心理震撼，是引发医疗纠纷的严重不良事件之一，对社会有着巨大的消极影响。在我国当前医患关系较为紧张的形势下，研究患者自杀问题，对减少医患纠纷、改善医患关系、提高医院声誉等具有重要的理论价值与实践意义。

　　医务人员要及时识别患者自杀征兆。自杀者在实施自杀前，往往会发出一些信号，只是周围的人并没有意识到。在自杀死亡的患者中，83%的患者在前一年向医院寻求过咨询，近50%的患者在前一个月向医院寻求过帮助，但得到精神心理健康诊断的患者仅占24%。临床一线医务人员作为直接接触患者的专业卫生保健人员，有必要认识并掌握患者自杀前言语与行为上的各种征兆，同时帮助患者及家属正确认识抑郁与自杀。

　　根据近30年来的自杀研究文献报告，国内对患者自杀的关注多集中于精神疾病患者。在我国自杀死亡者中，既往无精神障碍患者占40%；自杀未遂者中，既往无精神障碍患者占比高达60%。因此在我国患者自杀预防研究与实践中，不仅要关注精神障碍自杀风险患者，也需要重视和研究无精神障碍患者自杀预防问题。

　　事实证明，患者自杀是可以预防的。自杀由生物、心理、社会等综合因素导致，涉及多个领域，因此，需要多学科合作、多措并举共筑患者自杀预防防线。华中科技大学同济医学院附属协和医院"患者自杀预防"研究团队打破"禁区"，从患者自杀的理论研究到自杀预防干预的临床实践，对患者自杀风险管理进行了较为深入系统的研究，通过编译国外患者自杀风险管理相关共识指南，融合研究团队的思考与实践，形成了较为系统、全面的患者自杀风险管理体系并编制成指导手册。这是预防患者自杀研究迈出的一小步，也是我国医疗

1

机构预防患者自杀实践迈出的一大步，将充实丰富我国医疗机构临床实践服务内容，为医务人员实施患者自杀风险管理提供参考借鉴。

本书特色主要表现在以下几个方面：

（1）现实需求：住院患者存在一定的自杀风险，而大多数医务人员对患者自杀的认识尚且不足，本书介绍了自杀相关理论知识。（2）操作性强：本书介绍了患者自杀风险筛查、评估、预防与干预等实践建议，具有很强的实用价值。（3）内容全面：本书介绍了患者入院、住院期间、出院、随访全程的自杀风险管理过程以及文书记录管理等。同时，本书阐述了患者自杀风险管理基础、原则、方法、资源，为改善医务人员对预防患者自杀的态度、知识、能力提供最为直接可用的参考。

我们深信该书将会受到临床医务人员的欢迎，特在此郑重推荐。

北京大学回龙观临床医学院 北京心理危机研究与干预中心 童永胜
武汉大学人民医院 湖北省人民医院 郭 鑫
2021 年 2 月

前言

"自杀学"创始人爱米尔·迪尔凯姆将自杀定义为任何由死者自己完成并知道会产生这种结果的某种积极或消极行动直接或间接引起的死亡。为了引起公众对自杀的关注，2003年，世界卫生组织和国际预防自杀协会（IASP）将每年的9月10日定为"世界预防自杀日"。2003年9月10日是全球第一个"世界预防自杀日"，其主题为"自杀一个都太多"，表明了对预防自杀的决心和对生命的敬畏。中国医院协会结合当前医院质量与安全管理工作现状，制定了《患者安全目标》（2019版），目标六为防范与减少意外伤害，其中新增"识别具有自我攻击风险的患者，评估自我伤害、拒绝饮食、自杀倾向等行为，制定相应防范措施和应急处置预案"内容。卫生保健机构和医院是最有机会接触具有自杀风险患者的场所，因此，医务人员必须关注并提高对患者自杀意念和行为风险的识别与评估能力，预防和减少患者自杀行为的发生。

研究表明，患者自杀除了个体的生理、心理以及社会因素外，还可能与医院缺乏完善的患者自杀风险管理制度与实践有关。医院安全文化和管理制度直接或间接影响着患者的微观生存环境和生活质量，因此，提升医务人员患者自杀风险管理能力、培养预防患者自杀"守门人"势在必行。

华中科技大学同济医学院附属协和医院"患者自杀预防"研究团队关注并从事患者自杀预防研究近10年，研究发现，每一例患者自杀事件背后都有着令人心酸的故事。作为医务人员，在扼腕叹息之余，不禁思考：我们能否为那些徘徊在生死边缘的患者做些什么？如何做到对患者自杀倾向的早期发现和早期干预，防患于未然？

鉴于国内预防患者自杀的相关书籍比较匮乏，为弥补我国患者自杀预防理论与实践的不足，华中科技大学同济医学院附属协和医院"患者自杀预防"研究团队在国家自然科学基金面上项目的资助支持下，潜心学习国内外自杀预防相关知识，勤于实践，打破"禁区"，通过编译国外患者自杀预防相关内容，融合研究团队的思考与实践，形成了较为完善、系统的患者自杀风险管理体系并编制成指导手册，为患者生命保驾护航。

全书共分为五章。第一章为自杀风险患者护理概述，从自杀相关概念及定义着手，分析自杀流行病学特征，介绍自杀主要理论流派，提出了自杀风险管理原则、组织建议及实践建议。第二章为患者自杀风险评估，主要介绍患者自杀的影响因素、患者自杀风险评估流程及评估要素，从生理、心理、社会等多方面提出自杀风险患者的护理决策。第三章为患者自杀预防与干预，介绍了一些自杀预防和干预措施，帮助搭建以患者为中心的社会支持网络等。第四章为自杀风险患者的随访，通过介绍对自杀风险患者的随访，提供了实用性强、可操作性强的出院计划清单及社区资源清单模板。第五章为自杀风险患者的文书记录，为临床医务工作者护理自杀风险患者相关文书记录给出了参考意见。最后，本书以附录的形式简要介绍了常用自杀风险评估量表的使用、如何在法律允许的范围内分享患者健康信息并提供了关怀性联系样本资料等。全书内容深入浅出、言简意赅，旨在使广大读者深刻认识到预防患者自杀的重要性，并熟练掌握患者自杀风险管理的临床知识与相关技能。

感谢全体编写人员的智慧付出，感谢主审们的专业指导。预防患者自杀任重而道远，我们愿负重前行，因为我们有一个伟大的梦想——患者"零自杀"！研究团队将不忘初心、牢记使命，携手并肩、砥砺前行，重建患者希望，拯救患者生命！

本书适用于各级各类医院的医务人员，能够为预防患者自杀实践提供参考。由于时间仓促及经验有限，错误与不足之处敬请读者谅解与指正，以便再版时更正。

华中科技大学同济医学院附属协和医院

胡德英 刘义兰 孙晖

2021 年 2 月

目　　录

患者自杀风险管理指导手册（汉英对照）

1 自杀风险患者护理概述
1 Summary of Nursing Care for Suicide Risk Patients

1.1 自杀相关概念及定义
1.1 Related Concepts and Definitions of Suicide

自杀涉及心理学、社会学、伦理学、哲学、公共卫生等不同领域,由于自杀的复杂性,自杀相关概念缺乏普遍接受的标准化定义。自杀预防领域认为,自杀概念核心要素涉及自杀结果、行为中介、自杀意念水平以及对行为危险性的认识。

Suicide involves different fields such as psychology, sociology, ethics, philosophy, public health and so on. Suicide-related concepts also lack generally accepted standardized definitions due to their complexity. In the field of suicide prevention, the core elements of the concept of suicide involve suicide outcome, behavior mediation, level of suicide ideation and awareness of behavioral risk.

自杀术语的标准化经历了探索期、规范期、标准化期三个时期。探索期概念涵盖广泛,旨在提高自杀研究者之间沟通的清晰度和准确性。规范期不再追求概念的广泛性,旨在寻找自杀相关概念的核心特征。标准化期出现了哥伦比亚自杀评估分类法、国际疾病分类法。

The standardization of suicide terms has gone through three periods: exploration period, norming period and standardization period. The exploration period covers a wide range of subjects, aims to improve the clarity and accuracy of communication between suicide researchers. The norming period is no longer to pursue the broadness of the concept, aiming to find the core features of suicide-related concepts. During the standardization period, Columbia Classification Algorithmof Suicide Assessment and the International Classification of Diseases appeared.

世界卫生组织将自杀定义为故意杀死自己的行为,包括自杀意念、自杀计划、自杀未遂以及自杀死亡等一系列行为。我国学者肖水源根据我国国情将自杀主要分为自杀死亡、自杀未遂、自杀准备、自杀计划以及自杀意念。

The World Health Organization defines suicide as the act of deliberately killing oneself, including suicide ideation, suicide plans, attempted suicide, and committed suicide. According to China's national conditions, Xiao Shuiyuan, a Chinese scholar, divides suicide into committed suicide, attempted suicide, suicide preparation, suicide plan and suicide ideation.

自杀死亡即采取伤害自己生命的行为,且该行为直接导致了死亡的结局。自杀未遂即采取了伤害自己生命的行为,但该行为未直接导致死亡。自杀准备即做了自杀行为的准备如蓄药、购买自杀工具等,但未采取导致伤害生命的行为。自杀计划即有了明确伤害自己的计划,但没有实际准备,也没有采取任何实际行为。自杀意念即有了明确伤害自己的意愿,但没有形成自杀计划,没有做自杀行为的准备,也没有实际伤害自己的行为。

Committed suicide means taking actions to hurt one's own life, which directly leads to the outcome of death. Attempted suicide is an action that hurts one's life, but the action does not directly lead to death. Suicide preparation is the preparation of suicide behavior, such as storage of drugs, purchase of suicide tools, but did not take the behavior that leads to injury to life. The suicide plan means that there is a clear plan to hurt oneself, but there is no actual preparation action. Suicide ideation means that there is a clear intention to hurt oneself, but there is no plan for suicide, no behavioral preparation, and no actual action to hurt oneself.

自杀行为是个体在了解致命性行为后果的前提下,仍然采取某种致命性行为,以达到某种目的的过程。了解自杀相关概念及定义对临床评估、干预和医疗记录具有一定的指导意义。

Suicide behavior is a process in which individuals take certain fatal behaviors to achieve a certain purpose while they understand the consequences of fatal behaviors. Understanding suicide-related concepts and definitions has certain guiding significance for clinical evaluation, intervention and medical records.

1.2 自杀流行病学特征

1.2 Epidemiological Characteristics of Suicide

2015年,世界卫生组织报告称,自杀是15至29岁人群死亡的第二大原因。78%的自杀事件发生在中低收入国家,中国和印度的自杀人数占全球自杀总人数的30%。墨西哥、巴西、意大利、西班牙、英国、土耳其和新加坡等国家,自杀率在5.0%～9.9%之间。中国、加拿大、德国、葡萄牙和美国等国家,自杀率在10.0%～14.9%之间(Bachmann,2018)。

In 2015, the World Health Organization reported that suicide was the second leading cause of death among people aged 15 to 29. 78% of suicides occur in low-

and middle-income countries, and China and India account for 30% of global suicides. In countries such as Mexico, Brazil, Italy, Spain, the United Kingdom, Turkey and Singapore, the suicide rate is between 5.0% and 9.9%. In countries such as China, Canada, Germany, Portugal and the United States, the suicide rate is between 10.0% and 14.9%.

住院患者自杀是医院常见的前哨事件,综合医院的住院患者自杀率为1.8/10万~4.0/10万(Ang,2018)。躯体疾病患者是自杀的高危人群,尤其是不可治愈的或疼痛性的慢性疾病患者,在自杀死亡者中占25%~75%(邓云龙等,2014)。我国综合医院住院患者自杀发生率高,综合医院非精神卫生科住院病人自杀意念报告率为10.82%(孟艳君等,2020),自杀死亡者中有43%患有严重的躯体疾病。

Inpatient suicide is a common sentinel event in hospitals, and the suicide rate of inpatients in general hospitals is 1.8/100,000—4.0/100,000. Patients with physical diseases are a high-risk group for suicide, especially those with incurable or painful chronic diseases, accounting for 25%—75% of those who die by suicide. In China, the incidence of suicide among inpatients in general hospitals is high. The rate of suicide ideation of inpatients in non-psychiatric departments in general hospitals is 10.82%, and 43% of suicides suffer from serious physical diseases.

1.2.1 自杀方式
1.2.1 Suicide Method

自杀方法因国而异,最常见的方法是自缢、喝农药和使用火器。我国住院患者常见的自杀方法包括跳楼、刀具自杀、自缢和过量服药(胡德英,2018)。丁小萍等对湖北省45所综合医院非精神科住院患者自杀行为的调查研究显示,住院患者自杀主要发生在病房内,自杀方式以跳楼为主(丁小萍等,2019)。

Suicide methods vary from country to country, and the most common methods are hanging, drinking pesticides, using firearms. Common suicide methods for inpatients in China include jumping from the building, killing with a knife, hanging, and overdose. Ding Xiaoping et al. investigated the suicide behavior of inpatients from non-psychiatric departments in 45 general hospitals in Hubei Province. The suicide behavior of inpatients mainly occurred in wards, and the main suicide method was jumping from the building.

1.2.2 人群分布
1.2.2 Population Distribution

近年来,美国75岁以下各年龄组的自杀率有所上升,其中45~64岁成年人的自杀绝对增长率最大,从13.2/10万上升到19.2/10万(Stone et al.,2018)。在我国,年龄大于60岁的高龄者、低学历者、失业者、农民、慢性疾病及低自尊水平患者更易发生自杀行为。我国住院患者中,自杀女性多于自杀男性,农村居民自杀率高于城市居民(丁小萍等,2019)。

In recent years, the suicide rate of all age groups under the age of 75 in the United States has increased. Among them, the absolute growth rate of adults aged 45−64 years is the largest, rising from 13.2/100,000 to 19.2/100,000. In China, people aged over 60, with low education, unemployed, farmers, patients with chronic diseases and low self-esteem are more likely to commit suicide. There are more females commiting suicide than males in hospitalized patients in China and the suicide rate of rural residents is higher than that of urban residents.

1.2.3 自杀时间

1.2.3 Suicide Time

世界卫生组织报告显示,自杀意念在萌芽的第1年发展到自杀计划和自杀企图的可能性最大(崔黎黎等,2009)。国外研究显示,自杀未遂急诊就诊具有季节性特征,春季为高峰,初秋为小高峰,深秋或初冬为低谷(Canner et al.,2018)。我国学者对568例急诊科自杀未遂患者特征的分析显示,自杀行为多发生于春夏季,4～5月份最多(胡德英等,2018)。住院患者自杀行为多出现在春季、凌晨及住院1周以内(丁小萍等,2019)。

According to the World Health Organization, suicide ideation is most likely to develop into suicide plan and suicide attempt within the first year. Foreign studies show that emergency treatment for attempted suicide has seasonal characteristics, with the peak in spring, small peak in early autumn, and low in late autumn or early winter. An analysis of the characteristics of 568 suicide attempted patients in the emergency department by Chinese scholars shows that suicides mostly occur in spring and summer, with the most occuring in April and May. The suicide behaviors of hospitalized patients mostly occurred in spring, early morning and within one week after hospitalization.

1.2.4 自杀经济负担

1.2.4 Suicide Financial Burden

自杀行为除了对当事人造成痛苦外,对经济、社会也影响深重,这些影响包括治疗费用、卫生保健延续服务费用、公共卫生支出增加与劳动力参与率降低等。美国每年非致命性自残急诊的直接医疗费和误工费总计高达700亿美元(Stone et al.,2018)。

In addition to causing pain to the person concerned, suicide behavior has a profound impact on the economy and society, including treatment costs, health care continuing service costs, public health expenditures and reduced labor force participation rates. In the United States, the annual direct medical expenses and lost work fees for non-fatal self-harm emergency treatment total up to 70 billion dollars.

据我国学者徐东等粗略估算,我国每年由自杀导致的经济负担仅医疗费就高达35亿~40亿人民币(徐东等,2008)。毛世清等对我国湖北省某大型综合医院急诊科服毒自杀患者医疗费用分析的结果显示,226例服毒自杀患者中,口服农药者产生的医疗费用高达300万元。住院天数是影响医疗费用的主要因素(毛世清等,2020)。

According to rough estimates by Xu Dong, the economic burden of suicide every year in China is 3.5—4 billion RMB in medical expenses alone. Mao Shiqing *et al*. analysed medical expenses of suicide patients taking drugs in the emergency department of a large general hospital in Hubei Province. It shows that 226 cases of suicide patients taking pesticides incurred a total of 3 million yuan in medical expenses. The length of hospitalization is the main factor affecting the medical expenses.

1.3 自杀理论流派
1.3 Suicide Theory Sect

1.3.1 涂尔干的自杀论
1.3.1 Durkheim's Suicide Theory

法国社会学家涂尔干在其著作《自杀论》中对自杀现象进行了详细分析,并将自杀分为利己型自杀、利他型自杀、失范型自杀和宿命型自杀四种类型。自杀论同时还提到了代表社会凝聚力的社会整合和代表社会制约力的道德规范两种社会特征。其中,社会整合不足和社会整合过度分别会导致利己型自杀和利他型自杀。道德规范过宽和道德规范过严分别会导致失范型自杀和宿命型自杀。

French sociologist Durkheim analyzed suicide in detail in his book *Le Suicide*, and divided suicide into four types: egoistic suicide, altruistic suicide, anomic suicide and fatalistic suicide. The suicide theory also mentions two social characteristics: social integration representing social cohesion and moral norms representing social restraining force. Insufficient and excessive social integration will lead to egoistic suicide and altruistic suicide, respectively. Too broad and strict ethics will lead to anomie suicide and fatalistic suicide, respectively.

1.3.2 应激-易感理论
1.3.2 Stress-susceptibility Theory

Mann等提出了自杀的应激-易感模型,指出个体自杀意念的形成,首先必须具备自杀的特质型因素(如易感性、生物因素中的5-羟色胺功能紊乱、认知因素和人格特质),其次必须具备发展为自杀的状态型因素(如抑郁和焦虑、绝望感),自杀意念和自杀行为在触发因素如压力性事件等的作用下才会产生。自杀是易感因素、应激因素与保护性因素三者共同作用的过程(Mann et al.,2005)。

Mann et al. proposed a stress-susceptibility model of suicide, and pointed out that the formation of individual suicide ideation must first have suicide trait factors (such as susceptibility, biological factors of serotonin dysfunction, cognitive factors and personality traits). Second, it must have factors that develop into a suicide state (such as depression and anxiety, hopeless), and suicide ideation and behaviors can only occur under the influence of triggering factors such as stressful events. Suicide is a process in which susceptible factors, stress factors and protective factors work together.

1.3.3 自杀人际理论

1.3.3 The Suicide Interpersonal Theory

Joiner于2007年提出自杀人际理论。该理论认为,个人实施自杀行为需要具备以下三要素:归属受挫、累赘感知和习得的自杀能力。归属受挫指个人的人际需要未得到满足而产生的孤立感。累赘感知是社交能力没得到满足而产生的心理状态。归属受挫及累赘感知是个人产生自杀意念需要具备的两大要素。个体通过反复多次接触痛苦与刺激事件,可以降低对死亡的恐惧,并提高身体疼痛的容忍度,从而习得自杀能力。当个体同时具有归属受挫、累赘感知和习得的自杀能力时,就会实施自杀行为,甚至会导致自杀身亡。

Joiner put forward the suicide interpersonal theory in 2007. The theory states that individuals need three elements to commit suicide: thwarted belongingness, perceived burdensomeness and acquired capability for suicide. Thwarted belongingness refers to the sense of isolation that arises when an individual's interpersonal needs are not met. Perceived burdensomeness is a psychological state resulting from social competence not being satisfied. Thwarted belongingness and perceived burdensomeness are the two major elements needed to generate suicide ideation. Individuals can reduce the fear of death by repeatedly touching painful and stimulating events, and improve the tolerance of physical pain, so as to acquired capability for suicide. When an individual has thwarted belongingness, perceived burdensomeness and acquired capability for suicide at the same time, he/she will commit suicide which even leads to death.

1.3.4 自杀三阶段理论

1.3.4 The Three-Stage Theory of Suicide

Klonsky 和 May 在 2015 年提出了自杀三阶段理论,该理论认为个体从自杀意念到自杀企图经历了三个阶段。个体同时存在痛苦和绝望时会产生自杀意念,联结感使个体的自杀意念变得强烈或微弱。强烈的自杀意念在个体具有自杀能力的条件下会转变为自杀尝试行为。痛苦、绝望和联结感的交互作用影响自杀意念的强弱。个体是否有自杀能力是能否将自杀意念转化为自杀尝试行为的决定性因素。痛苦、绝望、联结感和自杀能力是自杀行为的核心成分。

Klonsky and May proposed the three-stage theory of suicide in 2015, which held that individuals have experienced three stages from suicide ideation to suicide attempt. When individuals have pain and hopelessness at the same time, they will generate suicide ideation. The connectedness makes the suicide ideation strong or weak. The strong suicide ideation will turn into suicide attempt when the individual has the ability to commit suicide. The interaction of pain, hopelessness and connectedness affect the strength of suicide ideation. Whether an individual has the ability to commit suicide is the decisive factor for whether the suicide idea can be transformed into suicide attempt. Pain, hopelessness, connectedness and capability for suicide are the core elements of suicide behavior.

1.3.5 自杀扭力理论

1.3.5 The Strain Theory of Suicide

国内学者张杰提出了自杀扭力理论。此理论认为自杀会由某一类不协调的压力引起。四种导致自杀不协调的压力分别是不同价值观的冲突、现实与愿望的冲突、相对剥夺、应对技能的缺乏。这些不协调的压力导致自杀过程还受到社会心理因素的调节影响以及心理病理学因素的强化影响。正是由于这两个中间因素的存在,大多数经历过不协调的压力的人并不会选择自杀。

Chinese scholar Zhang Jie proposed the strain theory of suicide. Suicide can be caused by a certain type of uncoordinated stress. The four types of uncoordinated pressures that lead to suicide are the conflict of different values, the conflict of reality and desire, relative deprivation, and the lack of coping skills. The process of suicide caused by these discordant stresses is also mediated by social psychosocial factors and reinforced by psychopathological factors. Because of the existence of these two intermediate factors, most people who experience uncoordinated pressure will not choose suicide.

1.4 自杀风险管理原则

1.4 Suicide Risk Management Principles

综合医院临床护理预防患者自杀工作主要遵循三个原则。①服务信念：通过服务质量的持续改进，可以消除住院患者的自杀意念。②系统管理：整合医疗社会资源，采取系统性干预计划。③循证临床护理实践：在护理系统中以高效的护患互动为重点，进行有针对性的循证临床干预。

The patients suicide prevention work of clinical nursing in general hospitals mainly follows three principles. ① Service belief：through continuous improvement of service quality, inpatients' suicide ideation can be eliminated.② System management：integrate medical social resources to adopt a systematic intervention strategy. ③ Evidence-based clinical nursing practice：focus on efficient nurse-patient interaction in the nursing system, and carry out targeted evidence-based clinical intervention.

评估和照顾有自杀意念和行为风险的成年人的指导原则包括以下内容：

Guiding principles in the assessment and care for adults at risk for suicide ideation and behaviour include：

①"精神病的耻辱感可以被定义为一种基于偏见和错误信息的消极态度，这种态度由疾病标志引发，例如行为异常或病历上提到精神病治疗"（Sartorius，2007）。"自杀耻辱感"同样可以被定义为一种基于偏见和错误信息的消极态度，这种态度是由自杀、自杀意念或自杀行为引起的。自杀、自杀意念和自杀行为有时与精神疾病有关。耻辱感的存在导致持续的偏见和边缘化，对患者、家庭和社区造成不利影响，这些影响包括自尊水平下降、孤立感和脆弱感增加，当患者有精神疾病史时，复发的可能性更高。

① "Stigma of mental illness can be defined as the negative attitude based on prejudice and misinformation that is triggered by a marker of illness-e.g., odd behaviour, or the mention of psychiatric treatment in a curriculum vitae". "Stigma of suicide" can be defined similarly as a negative attitude based on prejudice and misinformation that is triggered by suicide or suicide ideation or behaviour. Suicide, suicide ideation and behaviour is sometimes linked to a mental illness. The presence of stigma leads to ongoing discrimination and marginalization with detrimental effects for clients, families and communities of people, including decreased self-esteem, increased isolation and vulnerability and, in the presence of a mental illness, a higher probability of relapse.

②自杀是生命的突然终结,也是人们应对巨大痛苦最极端的方式。护士需要从患者的角度来理解这一点,并以一种非评判和非指责的方式对待这些行为。

②Suicide is an abrupt ending to life and the most extreme way in which people respond to overwhelming distress. The nurse needs to understand this from the perspective of the client and approach these actions in a non-judgmental and non-blaming way.

③当个体表现出自杀意念和自杀行为时,护士在干预中起着重要的作用。

③Nurses have a significant role in intervening when individuals express suicide ideation and behaviour.

④干预的目的是降低自杀意念和自杀行为的风险,并促进患者、工作人员和其他人的安全。护士不能阻止每一次自杀死亡。自杀是复杂的,自杀预防工作不能仅由少数人来完成。

④The goal of intervention is to reduce the risk of suicide ideation and behaviour, and to promote the safety of the client, staff and others. Nurses cannot stop every death by suicide. Suicide is complex, and prevention cannot rest solely in the hands of a small group of people.

⑤建立治疗性关系是这项工作的基础。

⑤Establishment of a therapeutic relationship is fundamental to this work.

⑥优秀的关系实践应考虑文化的差异和安全问题。

⑥Excellence in relational practice takes into consideration issues of difference and cultural safety.

⑦照顾有自杀意念和自杀风险的成年人,对护士有显著的心理和潜在的生理影响。工作环境必须为护士提供足够的支持。

⑦There are significantly psychological and potentially physical impacts on the nurse when providing care for adults at risk for suicide ideation and behaviour. The work environment must provide adequate supports for the nurse.

⑧在治疗计划中,护士应考虑支持心理健康和幸福的因素,同时牢记包括社会和文化因素在内的健康决定因素。支持内在的力量和自尊,提高压力管理所需的情绪应对能力和生活技能至关重要。

⑧In treatment planning, the nurse considers factors that support mental health and well being, keeping in mind determinants of health, including social and cultural factors. It is important to support internal strengths and self-esteem, and the development of emotional coping and life skills needed for stress management.

⑨当护士与跨学科团队、患者、家庭、社区合作时，最能实现安全、有效的护理。

⑨Safe, effective care is best achieved when nurses work in collaboration with the interdisciplinary team, client, family and community.

⑩文件是护理实践的标准，也是评估和护理有自杀意念和自杀行为风险患者的一个组成部分。

⑩Documentation is a standard of nursing practice and is an integral part of the assessment and care of clients at risk for suicidal ideation and behaviour.

1.5 自杀风险管理组织建议

1.5 Organizational Recommendations of Suicide Risk Management

建议1：接收自杀患者的医疗机构必须提供安全的物理环境，尽量减少自伤行为的途径。（Ⅳ类证据）

Recommendation 1：Health care organizations that admit suicidal clients must provide a safe physical environment that minimizes access to means for self-injurious behaviour.（Type Ⅳ Evidence）

接受自杀倾向患者的医疗机构必须提供一个安全的住院环境，尽量减少患者因建筑物的物理结构和构造获得自我伤害的机会（JCAHO，1998；Sullivan *et al.*，2005）。患者可能利用各种医疗物理环境结构，如门后挂衣钩、窗户、药物和化学物品作为自杀手段，因此，医疗机构需要确保住院环境、设施及设备的安全性。

Health care organizations that admit suicide clients must provide a physical environment that minimizes client access to methods within the physical architecture and structure of the building, whereby clients may harm themselves. Clients may utilize various structures of the physical health care environment, such as door hooks for clothing, windows, medications, and chemicals as methods for suicide behaviour. Therefore, organizations need to ensure that the physical environment, architecture and hardware are such that this potential is minimized.

减少环境对自杀患者的伤害的住院环境建议（JCAHO，1998；RCP，2006；Yeager *et al.*，2005）包括以下内容：

Suggested structural accommodations for the suicide client to diminish environmental harm are：

①使用承重力有限的构件,如挂钩。

②使用易打开和未设反锁结构的门。

③使用不易破碎且抗震的玻璃隔板。

④设置药物和有毒化学品安全区域。

⑤所有工作人员、后勤管理员和运输助理人员都要关注环境安全情况。

⑥设置紧急按钮,使用带有外部线路或其他紧急通信系统的电话。

① Using breakaway hardware, such as hooks.

② No doors cannot be opened easily by staff and are lockable inside.

③ Using non-breakable, shatterproof glass partitions.

④ Set up secure areas for medications and toxic chemicals.

⑤ All workers, housekeepers, and transport aides paying attention to safety in the environment.

⑥ Set up panic buttons, accessing telephones with an outside line or other emergency communication systems.

建议2:在接收自杀患者的医疗机构中,护理人员的补充应适应护患比例和人员组合(如注册护士、注册精神病学护士、护工),以安全地满足急性自杀患者不可预知的需求。(Ⅳ类证据)

Recommendation 2: In health care organizations that admit suicide patients, nursing staff complements should be appropriate to the nurse-to-patient ratio and to the staff proportion (i.e., RN, RPN, health care aide) to safely meet the unpredictable needs of acute suicide patients. (Type Ⅳ Evidence)

护士应能24小时随时联系急救人员,最好是精神科医生。护士在他们的工作中需要足够的时间来进行自杀风险评估,提供观察和监测,并满足患者的需要。如果可能,工作人员应反映当地自杀患者人群的年龄、性别和种族背景的综合情况(RCP,2006)。

Nurses should have 24-hour access to emergency personnel, preferably a psychiatrist. They require sufficient time in their workload to conduct suicide risk assessments, provide observation and monitoring, and meet the client's needs. If possible, the staff should reflect a mix of age, gender and ethnic backgrounds that reflect the local client population.

建议3:组织机构应确保系统地回顾有关自杀的重大事件,以找出在各级服务中学习的机会。(Ⅳ类证据)

Recommendation 3: Organizations should ensure that critical incidents involving suicide are reviewed systematically to identify opportunities for learning at all levels of service delivery. (Type Ⅳ Evidence)

组织必须确保所有医疗保健专业人员,在工作中按照指南实践,参与照顾有自杀意念和自杀风险的患者。许多因素都会影响病人在医疗机构方面的体验,以及随之而来的正面或负面健康结果。

Organizations must ensure that all health care professionals involved in providing care to adults at risk for suicide ideation and behaviour work in an environment that allows them to practice according to the guidelines. Many factors contribute to the client's experience with the health care system and the positive or negative health outcomes that follow.

当发生重大事件时,例如涉及自杀的事件,对可能导致事件发生的体系和过程问题进行分析,有助于找出学习的机会和质量改进计划的潜在目标(Dlugacz, *et al.*, 2003)。伦理决策框架可能有助于指导这一过程。

When a critical incident does occur, such as events involving suicide, an analysis of system and process issues that may have contributed to the incident can help identify opportunities for learning and potential targets for quality improvement initiatives. A framework for ethical decision-making may be helpful to guide this process.

建议4:各组织应在发生诸如自杀身亡的重大事件后,制定与同行汇报的有关政策和体系。制定支持工作人员和尽量减少替代性创伤的政策。(IV类证据)

Recommendation 4: Organizations should develop policies and structures related to peer debriefing following a critical incident, such as a death by suicide. Policies should be developed to support staff and minimize vicarious trauma. (Type IV Evidence)

在可能对工作人员产生负面影响的重大事件发生后,各组织必须积极为需要咨询或支持的个人提供适当的服务。同行汇报可能是满足这一需要的一种方法。有关同行汇报的详细资料,请参阅实践建议部分。

Organizations must take an active role in making appropriate services available for individuals in need of counseling or support following critical incidents that may have negative impact on staff. Peer debriefing may be one method by which this need may be met. For further details regarding peer debriefing, please refer to the Practice Recommendations section.

替代性创伤,也称为继发性创伤反应,是指帮助过创伤事件受害者的人所经历的心理后遗症(Varcarolis, 2002)。

Vicarious traumatization, also known as a secondary trauma response, is a condition in which psychological aftereffects are experienced by those who assist victims of traumatic events.

建议5:各组织分配资源时,应确保所有护士均有机会获得持续的临床督导和辅导。(Ⅳ类证据)

Recommendation 5: Organizations should allocate resources to ensure that all nurses have opportunities for clinical supervision and coaching on an ongoing basis. (Type Ⅳ Evidence)

即使在没有重大事件的情况下,持续的临床督导和指导仍可帮助降低对护士产生负面影响的可能性,并促进临床技能的提高(NZGG,2003;RNAO,2006b)。要做到这一点,各组织必须分配财政资源,以支付临床督导和指导费用,并确保配备包括高级护士在内的人员组合,这可以帮助其他护士确定自己的专业优势和不足。

Even in the absence of critical events, clinical supervision and coaching on an ongoing basis may help to mitigate the potential for negative impacts to the nurse, as well as promote the refinement of clinical skills. To accomplish this, organizations must allocate financial resources to cover the cost of clinical supervision and coaching, and ensure a staffing mix that includes senior nurses who can help other nurses to identify their own professional strengths and weaknesses.

这样的高级护士需要有经验、接受过教育并有能力进行客观的自我评价。如果临床监督是由一名对其没有行政管理权力的护士提供的,这一过程将得到加强(RNAO,2006b)。关于临床监督的更多细节,请参考建议13。

Such a senior nurse needs to have experience, education, and the ability to facilitate objective self-evaluation. This process is enhanced if the clinical supervision is provided by a nurse with no administrative authority over the senior nurse. For further details regarding clinical supervision, please refer to Recommendation 13.

建议6:各组织应实施有关系统记录自杀风险评估的策略。(Ⅳ类证据)

Recommendation 6: Organizations should implement policies regarding the systematic documentation of suicide risk assessments. (Type Ⅳ Evidence)

虽然在记录自杀风险评估的标准方法上没有达成共识,但这一指南建议各组织制定政策,确保采取系统的措施。自杀风险评估的有效沟通是促进适当照护患者的基础(Sullivan *et al.*,2005)。NZGG(2003)还强调了结构化评估的重要性,它可以避免关键的评估信息被忽视。

Although there is no consensus on a standard way to document suicide risk assessments, this guideline recommends that organizations develop policies to ensure that a systematic process is adopted. Effective communication of suicide risk assessments is fundamental to promoting appropriate care for the client (Sullivan *et al.*, 2005). The NZGG (2003) also emphasize the importance of a structured assessment as a way to avoid having key assessment information overlooked.

一份描述性研究显示,确定文件系统结构的政策与社会心理评估的充分性增加有关(Crawford *et al.*, 1998)。记录评估信息的一致过程也有利于收集有价值的数据,以供评价和质量监测之用(Hawton *et al.*, 2006; Horrocks, House, and Owens, 2004)。

In one descriptive study, a policy that identifies a systematic structure for documentation was associated with increased adequacy of psychosocial assessment. A consistent process for documenting assessment information may also lead to the collection of valuable data for evaluation and quality monitoring purposes.

建议7:各组织应在组织和社区内推广可用的服务,这些服务可能会对有自杀意念和自杀风险行为的成人提供支持。(IV类证据)

Recommendation 7: Organizations promote the services available within the organization and community that may support the care of adults at risk for suicide ideation and behaviour. (Type IV Evidence)

照顾有自杀意念和自杀行为风险的患者,需要多学科小组在延续护理中协调合作。为了适当和有效地利用现有资源,护士必须通过服务之间的联系得到支持。建议各组织在内部开展工作(即建立一个专门的评估小组),并与社区合作者共同制定延续护理的协作和一体化战略。

The care of individuals at risk for suicide ideation and behaviour requires a coordinated effort by the multidisciplinary team across the continuum of care. In order to appropriately and effectively utilize all available resources, the nurse must be supported through existing linkages between services. It is recommended that organizations work both internally (i.e., with the development of a specialized assessment team) and with community partners to develop strategies for collaboration and integration across the continuum of care.

服务计划小组需要包括多专业成员,包括紧急顾问、精神科专家、社会工作人员、用户团体代表和当地社区机构。如果可能,代表应具有不同的背景(RCP, 2004)。

Service planning groups need to include a multi-professional membership including emergency consultants, psychiatric specialists, social workers, representatives of user groups and local community agencies. If possible, representatives should be of diverse backgrounds.

建议8：各机构应支持护士在心理健康护理方面的专业发展机会。(Ⅳ类证据)

Recommendation 8: Organizations should support nurses' opportunities for professional development in mental health nursing. (Type Ⅳ Evidence)

卫生保健组织和学术机构必须合作，确保护士具备核心能力，以照顾有自杀意念和自杀风险者在内的心理健康需要者(Barling and Brown, 2001)。

Health care organizations and academic institutions must work collaboratively to ensure that nurses are equipped with the core competencies to care for individuals with mental health needs, including those who are at risk for suicide ideation and behaviour.

建议9：各组织应支持有关自杀和其他心理健康问题的研究项目。(Ⅳ类证据)

Recommendation 9: Organizations should support research initiatives related to suicide and other mental health issues. (Type Ⅳ Evidence)

为了更好地了解有效的护理方法，必须支持有关降低自杀风险和预防自杀风险的护理研究，从而加强现有的证据基础，以指导临床和管理层面的决策。

Nursing research related to suicide risk reduction and prevention must be supported in order to have better understanding of effective approaches for care, and therefore to strengthen the evidence base available on which to guide decision-making both at clinical and administrative levels.

建议10：各组织应制定执行最佳实践指南建议的计划。(Ⅳ类证据)

Recommendation 10: Organizations should develop a plan for the implementation of best practice guideline recommendations. (Type Ⅳ Evidence)

①对组织准备状况和教育障碍的评估。

②所有对实施进程作出贡献的成员(无论是发挥直接或间接的支持作用)全部参与。

③不断提供讨论和教育的机会，以加强最佳实践的重要性。

④专业人员为教育和执行过程提供所需便利的献身精神。

⑤反思个人和组织在执行指导方针方面的经验的机会。

⑥可持续性战略。

⑦为执行可持续性发展分配足够的资源，包括组织和行政支持。

①An assessment of organizational readiness and barriers to education.

②Involvement of all members（whether in a direct or indirect supportive function）who will contribute to the implementation process.

③Ongoing opportunities for discussion and education to reinforce the importance of best practices.

④Dedication of a qualified individual to provide the facilitation required for the education and implementation process.

⑤Opportunities for reflection on personal and organizational experience in implementing guidelines.

⑥Strategies for sustainability.

⑦Allocation of adequate resources for implementation and sustainability, including organizational and administrative support.

执行指南的一个关键步骤是必须正式采纳和评价指南。各组织需要考虑如何将所采纳的建议正式纳入其政策和程序结构（Graham *et al.*, 2002）。正式采纳是将准则纳入现有的政策和程序。这一首要步骤为指南的普遍接受和整合到质量管理等系统中奠定了基础。

A critical initial step in the implementation of guidelines must be the formal adoption and evaluation of the guidelines. Organizations need to consider how to formally incorporate the recommendations to be adopted into their policy and procedure structure. An example of such a formal adoption would be the integration of the guideline into existing policies and procedures. This initial step paves the way for general acceptance and integration of the guideline into such systems as the quality management process.

1.6 自杀风险管理实践建议

1.6 Practice Recommendations of Suicide Risk Management

建议1：护士应认真对待患者直接或间接表示希望自杀的陈述和表明有自杀风险的所有可获得信息。（Ⅲ类证据）

Recommendation 1: The nurse should take seriously all statements made by the client that indicate, directly or indirectly, a wish to die by suicide, and all available information that indicates a risk for suicide. (Type Ⅲ Evidence)

有时，间接表达是行为上的而不是口头上的，例如储存药物、拟定遗嘱、安排葬礼、解决财产问题、捐赠财物、为科学捐献遗体、忽略关心自己或人际关系、在宗教信仰方面较平常有或多或少的改变、健康状况恶化(Holkup,2002)。

Sometimes the indirect expression is behavioural rather than verbal, such as storing medications, making a will, arranging for a funeral, settling financial affairs, giving belongings away, donating body to science, neglecting to care for self or relationships, sudden changes in religiosity-either greater or less than usual, or a deterioration in health.

此外,特别是对老年人而言,人们给出的指标可能是躯体性的。自杀死亡者在死亡前数周因疼痛等身体不适去看医生的情况并不少见(Holkup,2002)。关于预警信号和危险因素的详细资料,请参阅建议6。

Furthermore, the indicators that people give may be somatic in nature, particularly with elderly people. It is not uncommon for people who die by suicide to have been to a health care clinician weeks prior to their death for physical complaints, such as pain. Refer to Recommendation 6 for a more detailed description of warning signs and risk factors.

患者状况应该被认为是潜在的紧急情况,直到临床医生进行了其他评估(NZGG,2003)。"认真对待"还包括对一系列社会状况(如亲人的突然离世)和情绪状态(如抑郁)的敏感性认识,这些因素的合并增加了自杀风险(APA,2003;Holkup,2002)。

The client's status should be considered a potential emergency until assessed otherwise by clinicians. "Taking seriously" also includes being sensitive to, and aware of, the constellation of social situations such as sudden losses, and emotional states such as depression, that combine to increase the risk factors for suicide.

众所周知,自杀死亡者往往有自伤史,因此我们也应该认真对待那些没有表达死亡愿望的自伤意图和行为。此外,自伤和自杀行为者在不同的场合可能有不同的意图,因此,对每一事件都要给予充分的尊重和照顾(APA,2003;Royal College of Psychiatrists,2004)。

Self-harm intentions and behaviours without the expressed desire to die should also be taken seriously, as it is known that people who die by suicide frequently have had previous self-harm attempts. Also, people who engage in self-harm and suicidal behaviour may have different intentions on different occasions and therefore, each event is to be treated with full respect and care.

反复发生自伤行为的人往往低估了其自伤行为的致命性。每一次自伤事件都必须评估其致命性及采取相应的护理措施,不能被弱化或轻视。自杀可能在没有预兆的情况下发生，且带有冲动性。即使尽最大的努力，自杀也不可能总是得到预防。然而，护士有法律和道德上的责任尽可能防止患者自杀（Royal Australian and New Zealand College of Psychiatrists Clinical Practice Guidelines Team for Deliberate Self-harm，2004）。

People who engage in repeated episodes of self-harm behaviour may underestimate the lethality of their behaviour. Each episode of self-harm must be assessed for lethality and care needs to be taken that self-harm events are not minimized or trivialized. Suicide can occur without warning and be impulsive in nature. Even with best efforts, suicide cannot always be prevented. However, nurses have a legal and ethical responsibility to try to prevent a suicide where possible.

实践框

Practice Box

"认真对待"

"Taking seriously"

（RNAO Development Panel， 2008）

①所有可能表达死亡的言语和非言语行为都应被认真对待。

②评估患者的自杀风险。

　以下是询问患者是否有自杀倾向的一些建议：

　　■ "你在考虑结束你的生命吗？"

　　■ "你想自杀吗？"

　　■ "你有计划自杀吗"

　　■ "你是否有过死亡或自杀的想法？"

③评估结果记录在案，并传达给卫生保健小组的适当成员。

④在评估的基础上，采取适当的干预措施。

Ⅳ 类证据

①All verbal and non-verbal behaviours that may convey an expression of dying are taken seriously.

②The client is assessed for suicide risk.

Here are some suggestions to ask your client if he/she is suicidal：

　　■ "Are you thinking about ending your life?"

　　■ "Are you suicidal?"

　　■ "Do you have a plan to take your own life?"

　　■ "Do thoughts of death or suicide enter your mind?"

③The assessment is documented and communicated to the appropriate members of the health care team.

④Based upon the assessment， appropriate interventions are initiated.

Type Ⅳ Evidence

建议2：护士应致力于与有自杀意念和自杀行为风险的患者建立治疗关系。

（Ⅳ 类证据）

Recommendation 2: The nurse should work toward establishing a therapeutic relationship with clients at risk for suicide ideation and behaviour. (Type Ⅳ Evidence)

重要的是,护士必须认识到特殊情况可能会增加建立治疗关系的困难。患者的某些特征(如异常激动)可能会增加其参与治疗关系的难度。促进安全的干预措施,如呼叫紧急服务或提高观察等级,可能会被患者认为破坏了护患之间的信任,因此这是另一种潜在的挑战。

Importantly, the nurse must acknowledge that particular circumstances may pose challenges to the establishment of a therapeutic relationship. Certain client characteristics (e.g., if the client is highly agitated), may make engagement in a therapeutic relationship especially difficult. Interventions to promote safety, such as calling emergency services or increasing the level of observation, may be perceived by the client to be a breach of trust, and therefore represent another potential challenge.

此外,护士自身对死亡和自杀的态度会对建立治疗关系构成障碍,消极情绪的激活会引发护士的防御反应(APA, 2003),从而影响其建立治疗关系的能力。

Moreover, the nurse's own feelings toward death and suicide can pose an obstacle itself; the activation of these emotions may lead to defensive responses on the part of the nurse, thereby impacting one's ability to establish a therapeutic relationship.

这些充满挑战性的情景以及移情和反移情的问题,都需要合作、指导和临床督导,来帮助护士建立一种对患者的治疗性关系,并且培养护士的自我意识感。

Working through these challenging situations, as well as issues of transference and counter-transference, requires collaboration, mentorship and clinical supervision, all of which support the nurse in establishing a relationship that is therapeutic for the client and developing a sense of self-awareness regarding her or his practice.

有关治疗性关系的更多信息,请参阅 RNAO 最佳实践指南:建立治疗关系(已修订)(RNAO, 2006c)。

For more information regarding therapeutic relationships, refer to the RNAO Best Practice Guideline: Establishing Therapeutic Relationships (Revised).

建议3:护士应与患者合作,尽量减少与其自杀、精神疾病和成瘾有关的羞耻感、罪恶感和耻辱感。(Ⅲ类证据)

Recommendation 3: The nurse should work with the client to minimize the feelings of shame, guilt and stigma that may be associated with suicidality, mental illness and addiction. (Type Ⅲ Evidence)

自杀在当代社会一直受到指责(Murray and Hauenstein, 2008),这对有自杀想法和自杀行为风险的个体产生了影响。羞耻感、负罪感和耻辱感对患者的心理健康、家庭和社会支持系统、专业帮助和咨询的获取以及对他们的自尊都有累积性的影响(Barlow and Morrison, 2002; Ostman and Kiellin, 2002)。

Suicide continues to be stigmatized in contemporary society, leading to implications for individuals at risk for suicide ideation and behaviour. Feelings of shame, guilt and stigma have an accumulative effect on clients' mental well-being, on their families and social support system, on accessing professional help and counseling, and on their self-esteem.

一项研究发现,患者自杀未遂之后通常会有羞耻反应(Wiklander, Samuelsson, and Asberg, 2003)。在治疗性关系中,尊重、宽容和对患者自我价值肯定的表达可能有助于将这些感受降到最低(Ashmore, 2001; Wiklander *et al.*, 2003)。Wiklander 和他的同事(2003)认为在这种环境中,自杀患者羞耻感会减少,更愿意接受治疗。

One study found that suicide attempts are commonly followed by shame reactions. Within the therapeutic relationship, expressions of respect, tolerance and an affirmation of the client's self-worth may help to minimize these feelings. Wiklander and his colleagues (2003) suggest that suicide clients accept treatment better and feel less ashamed in such environments.

当护士没有急切想了解患者创伤性生活事件的细节时,患者同样会受益(NZGG, 2003)。此外,一项研究报告称,减少指责能大幅度降低美国空军人员自杀率(Knox *et al.*, as cited in Sakinofsky, 2007b)。为了最大限度地减少护士自身对患者潜在负面反应的影响,护士应进行反思实践并获得支持来应对这些挑战,这是至关重要的(McMain, 2007)。

Clients may benefit similarly when not pushed for traumatic life event details by the nurse. Moreover, one study reported that the reduction of stigmatization proved critical in declining suicidality in US Air Force personnel. To minimize the effect of the nurse's own potentially negative reactions to the client, it is essential that nurses engage in reflective practice and obtain support to address such challenges.

医护人员应注意自身的消极态度、信念和行为,它们可能会对患者产生负面影响。

Beware of your own negative attitudes, beliefs and behaviours, which may have negative impact on the client.

建议4：护士提供护理应遵循文化安全/文化能力的原则。（Ⅲ类证据）

Recommendation 4：The nurse should provide care in keeping with the principles of cultural safety/cultural competence. (Type Ⅲ Evidence)

患者和护士在治疗关系中，都会有他们自己的文化观、价值观和信念。因此，在这种关系的背景下，文化可能极大地影响双方对心理健康、自杀和死亡等问题的讨论和处理。例如，文化可能影响自杀产生的愧疚感和羞耻感（NZGG，2003；Proctor，2005），谈论死亡和自杀的意愿（APA，2003），以及家庭和社区在提供照料方面的态度（NZGG，2003）。

Both the client and nurse bring their own culturally derived attitudes, values and beliefs to the therapeutic relationship. As such, culture can greatly impact how issues of mental health, suicide and death are discussed and addressed in the context of this relationship. For example, culture may influence feelings of guilt and shame regarding suicide, the willingness to speak about death and suicide, and attitudes regarding family and community roles in care provision.

医疗服务提供者在患者的健康上扮演着重要的角色，医护人员和患者之间的文化差异可能会恶化这种关系，这对患者的护理经历以及临床实践的有效性和安全性都产生影响。

Health care providers have a powerful role in the health of the client, and cultural differences between the nurse and client may exacerbate these power relations. This has implications on the client's experience of care as well as the effectiveness and safety of clinical practice.

从批判的文化角度看，文化是复杂的、动态的、政治的、历史的——这是一个随着时间推移而变化的关系过程，"取决于我们的历史、过去的经历和我们的社会、职业和性别，以及我们如何看待社会对我们自身的看法"（Browne and Varcoe，2006）。

From a critical cultural perspective, culture is complex, dynamic, political and historical—it is a relational process that shifts over time "depending on our history, our past experiences, our social, professional and gendered location, and our perceptions of how we are viewed in society".

文化安全是新西兰奥特雅瓦罗的护士在护理教育中提出的一个概念（Ramsden，1993；2000）。其护士认识到，由于持续的殖民过程，毛利人在健康状况和保健方面存在不平等。文化安全始于护士/医疗服务提供者的自我反省。护士需要认识到患者（作为个人、家庭和/或社区）和提供者都是文化的承担者，总是1对1的"二元文化"关系。

Cultural safety is a concept which began in nursing education in Aotearoa, New

Zealand with Maori nurses in recognition of inequities in health status and health care for Maori related to continuing colonizing processes and practices. Cultural safety begins with the self-reflection of the nurse/ health care provider. The nurse needs to recognize that both the client (as individual, family and/or community) and the provider are "bearers of culture"—a 1:1 relationship is always bicultural.

它需要考查每个人在影响医疗保健、健康和福祉的历史、社会、经济和政治进程中的地位;认识到医疗保健中权力地位的差异会影响健康和福祉,需要加以解决;认识到影响保健、健康和福祉的结构性不平等现象需要按照护理的社会使命进行转变(Ramsden, 1993)。

It requires an examination of how each individual is located within historical, social, economic and political processes that influence health care, health and well-being; an understanding that differential positions of power in health care that influence health and well-being need to be addressed; and a recognition that structural inequities that impact health care, health and well-being need to be shifted in keeping with the social mandate of nursing.

文化安全不仅仅是承认和尊重"差异"——这是一个关系概念,需要参与影响保健和健康的政策和实践。护士表示要接受和尊重患者的"文化"和相关差异,并倡导改变患者可能经历的"不安全"的政策和做法。

Cultural safety is more than recognizing and respecting "difference"—it is a relational concept that demands engagement with policies and practices that impact health care and health. The nurse demonstrates acceptance and respect for the "culture" of the client and for the associated differences, in addition to advocating for change in response to policies and practices that may be experienced as "unsafe" by the client.

建议 5:护士应评估和管理可能影响患者和跨学科团队人身安全的因素。(Ⅳ类证据)

Recommendation 5: The nurse should assess and manage factors that may impact the physical safety of both the client and the interdisciplinary team. (Type Ⅳ Evidence)

在实施干预以增强病人的安全前,护士应先确保自己的安全。这可能包括寻求其他人的帮助,如团队成员、警察,甚至离开现场,直到得到适当的帮助。

Before intervening to enhance the client's safety, the nurse needs to ensure her/his own safety first. This may involve enlisting the help of others, such as team members, police, or even leaving the scene until appropriate supports are in place.

在提供护理时,照顾患者的人身安全是一个持续的优先事项,应在完成对自杀风险的全面临床评估之前启动。根据不同的实践环境,干预措施有很大的不同,虽然它们不能保证自伤行为不会发生,但这些干预措施可以最大限度地减少这种行为对患者和医疗团队的身体威胁。

Attending to the physical safety of the client is an ongoing priority when providing nursing care and should be initiated before a thorough clinical assessment of suicide risk is completed. Interventions are highly variable depending on the practice setting, and though they may not guarantee that self-injurious actions will not occur, these interventions may minimize the physical threat of such behaviour on the client and health care team.

为了与治疗关系保持一致,在实施安全措施的整个过程中,必须让患者和家属参与进来。护士应警惕物理环境和任何可能对安全构成威胁的物品。在适当的情况下,将这些物品从医院病房或家中移除。

In keeping with the therapeutic relationship, it is imperative to engage the client and family throughout the process of implementing safety measures. The nurse should be alert to the physical setting and any item in it that may pose a threat to safety. Reduce access by removing such items from the person and the environment, be it the hospital room or the home, as appropriate.

虽然没有防自杀病房,但鼓励医疗机构设置可能对自杀意念和自杀行为的患者有效的物理安全设施(Simon, 2004; Yeager et al., 2005)。也有人认为,外界的刺激如噪音和喧闹,可能会增加躁动和攻击性(Joint Commission on Accreditation of Healthcare Organizations, 1998)。在这种情况下,减少刺激源或将患者转移到刺激较小的环境可能是有帮助的。

Though there is no such thing as a suicide-proof unit, physical safety features are encouraged for organization-based settings that may potentially work with clients at risk for suicide ideation and behaviour. It is also suggested that external stimuli, such as noise and commotion, may increase agitation and aggression. In such cases, reducing the cause of stimuli or moving to a less stressful area may be helpful.

在某些情况下,患者可能会出现需要医疗照顾的身体伤害,危及生命的伤害应立即处理。同时不应低估其他伤害的严重性,并在评估患者护理需要时优先考虑(National Collaborating Centre for Mental Health , 2004)。在这种情况下,有必要进行持续的医疗和身体评估。

In some cases, the client may present with physical injury that requires medical attention. Life threatening injuries should be addressed immediately. The acuity of other injuries should not be underestimated and should be considered when prioritizing the client's care needs. Ongoing medical and physical assessment is warranted in such cases.

维护患者的尊严是至关重要的。情感和心理安全的考虑应与确保人身安全相平衡。例如,限制性干预,如隔离或限制,虽然有时在住院环境中使用以维护安全,但也可能对患者造成了很大压力,这种通过加强失控的感觉阻碍了患者康复(Murray and Hauenstein, 2008)。

Maintaining the client's dignity is essential. Considerations of emotional and psychological safety should be balanced with ensuring physical safety. For example, restrictive interventions, such as seclusion or restraints, although sometimes used in inpatient settings to maintain safety, may also be very stressful for clients and hinder recovery by reinforcing perceptions of being out of control.

因此,在实施任何安全措施时,让患者了解并参与决策过程很重要。

Therefore, when any safety measures are implemented, it is important to keep the client informed and engaged in the decision-making process.

实践框

潜在危险的物品可能包括,但不限于(Bennett *et al.*, 2006):

衣物(如腰带,鞋带)	其他设备
绳索	氧疗装置和管道
打火机	塑料袋
亚麻布	锋利的或玻璃的物体
药物	有毒物质

Ⅳ类证据

Practice Box

Potentially hazardous items may include, but are not limited to:

clothing (e.g., belts, shoelaces)	other equipment
cords	oxygen therapy devices and tubing
lighters	plastic bags
linens	sharp or glass objects
medications	toxic substances

Type Ⅳ Evidence

建议 6a:护士应认识到,即使在没有明确自杀倾向的情况下,也有使个体发生自杀行为的关键指标。对于表现出风险指标的个体,护士应对其自杀意念和自杀计划进行评估和记录。(Ⅳ类证据)

Recommendation 6a: The nurse should recognize key indicators that put an individual at risk for suicidal behaviour, even in the absence of expressed suicidality. For individuals who exhibit risk indicators, the nurse should conduct and document an assessment of suicide ideation and plan. (Type Ⅳ Evidence)

总的来说,通过与卫生保健小组合作,使用临床判断来决定风险评估和重新评估的频率。如果护士怀疑患者有自杀意念和自杀行为的风险,则需要进一步评估患者的自杀意念和自杀计划。

Overall, the estimation of risk and decisions regarding the frequency of reassessment is best conducted through the use of clinical judgment, in collaboration with the health care team. If the nurse suspects a risk of suicide ideation and behaviour, then further assessment of the suicide ideation and plan is required.

没有证据表明直接询问自杀会增加自杀意念和自杀行为的可能性(APA,2003;NZGG,2003)。根据 APA(2003),"询问自杀是必要的,不会导致自杀"。评估与自杀有关的因素有助于揭示自杀想法和自杀行为背后的目的和意义,从而有助于制定适当的、有意义的干预措施(Murray and Hauenstein,2008)。

There is no evidence to suggest that asking a person directly about the topic of suicide will increase the likelihood of suicide ideation and behaviour. According to APA (2003), "Asking about suicide is necessary and will not lead the person to suicide". An assessment specific to factors related to suicide helps to uncover the purpose and meaning behind any suicide ideation and behaviour, thereby informing the

25

development of appropriate and meaningful interventions.

实践框

Practice Box

访谈举例

来源：NZGG（2003）.

Example interview questions

Source：NZGG（2003）.

■你最近心情如何？

■你有什么麻烦或担心吗？

■你曾经有过悲伤或沮丧的时候吗？

■你有觉得生活凌驾于你之上吗？

■你是否有时候希望你能让一切都停止，或是干脆结束这一切吗？

■你有没有想过该怎么做？

■你有没有希望自己死去？

■你想过结束自己的生命吗？

■How has your mood been lately?

■Has anything been troubling or worrying you?

■Have you had times when you have been feeling sad or "down"?

■Have you ever felt like life is just getting on top of you?

■Do you sometimes wish you could just make it all stop, or that you could just end it?

■Have you thought about how you might do this?

■Have you ever wished you were dead?

■Have you ever thought about taking your own life?

Ⅳ 类证据

Type Ⅳ Evidence

为全面评估自杀意念及自杀计划,可利用临床访谈及使用有效且可靠的评估工具搜集以下资料（APA，2003；NZGG，2003）：

To conduct a comprehensive assessment regarding suicide ideation and plan, a clinical interview and use of valid and reliable assessment tools may be used to gather information specific to:

• 存在危险因素；

• 缺乏或存在保护因素（例如精神、希望、未来方向、文化或精神因素）；

• 自杀意念；

• 计划；

• 致命性；

• 获得手段；

• 时间表；

• 希望；

• 自杀未遂。

• presence of risk factors；

• lack or presence of protective factors (e.g., spirituality, hope, future orientation, cultural or spiritual factors)；

• suicidal ideation；

• plan；

• lethality；

• access to means；

• timeframe；

• hope；

• suicide attempted.

对护士来说，参与有关自杀的讨论是很困难的。虽然团队合作和临床监督可能是护士在这些情况下获得支持的方式，但同样重要的是，护士必须具备适当的技能和知识水平，才能以治疗的方式进行这些临床评估。

Engaging in discussions regarding suicide can be difficult for the nurse. While teamwork and clinical supervision may be means by which a nurse may acquire support through these situations, it is also important to note that nurses must have the appropriate level of skill and knowledge to conduct these clinical assessments in a therapeutic way.

评估工具只能作为综合评估的一部分使用，且不应独立使用（APA，2003；NZGG，2003）。尽管种类繁多，但支持使用任何特定工具的证据有限。此外，现有的工具在判断个体是否会死于自杀的预测能力很低（APA，2003）。

Assessment tools are only to be used as part of a comprehensive assessment and should not be used in isolation. Despite the wide variety, there is limited evidence to support the use of any particular tool. Moreover, existing tools have low predictive ability to determine who will or will not die by suicide.

因此，这一指南表明，虽然这些工具可能有助于在访谈的范围内促进交流和信息收集，但这些结果并不能取代实践机构的临床判断。心理量表评估应留给经过专门培训的医护人员使用。

As such, this guideline suggests that while these tools may help to facilitate communication and information gathering in the context of an interview, the results do not replace clinical judgment in the practice setting. The use of psychological scales for diagnosis should be reserved for clinicians with specialized training.

特别考虑：中毒

Special Consideration: Intoxication

当患者中毒时，要进行全面的自杀风险评估是非常困难的。在这种情况下，评估应侧重于自杀的直接风险，而中毒的患者应被安置在安全的环境中，并在其清醒时重新评估（NZGG，2003）。同时还应评估中毒患者与药物使用有关的即时医疗问题。

When the presenting client is intoxicated, it can be extremely difficult to conduct a comprehensive suicide risk assessment. In such cases, assessment should focus on immediate risk for suicide and the intoxicated client should be kept in a safe environment and reassessed when sober. Individuals presenting with intoxication should also be assessed for immediate medical concerns related to the substance use.

例如，根据已建立的协议，有必要对那些已知或怀疑经常饮酒的人进行戒断症状的持续评估和管理（即潜在的酒精性癫痫发作，震颤性谵妄）。持续的医疗评估联合自杀风险评估对维护患者的安全至关重要。

For example, in those known or suspected to frequent use of alcohol, it is necessary to provide ongoing assessment and management of symptoms of withdrawal (i.e., potential alcohol-related seizures, Delirium Tremens), according to established protocols. Ongoing medical assessment in conjunction with assessment of suicide risk is essential to maintaining the safety of the client.

中毒（如酒精、诱导药物、多重用药、非处方药等）可能会增加冲动（NZGG，2003），因此强化了保护中毒和自杀意念的个人安全的必要性。根据新西兰指南（2003），中毒也可能增加人的痛苦、侵略性和降低解决问题的能力。

Intoxication (e.g., from alcohol, elicit drugs, polypharmacy, over-the-counter drugs, etc.) may increase impulsivity, and therefore reinforces the need to keep individuals presenting with intoxication and suicidal ideation safe. According to the New Zealand guidelines, intoxication may also increase the person's distress, aggressiveness and decrease problem-solving abilities.

此外，有证据表明，酗酒/中毒是自杀未遂的一个常见前奏（APA，2003）。持续评估自杀风险是至关重要的。

Moreover, evidence demonstrates that alcohol use/intoxication is a common prelude to a suicide attempt. Ongoing assessment of suicide risk is essential.

建议6b：护士应评估与自杀预防有关的保护因素。（Ⅳ类证据）

Recommendation 6b: The nurse should assess for protective factors associated with suicide prevention. (Type Ⅳ Evidence)

NZGG（2003）定义保护因素为"一个人生活中给予他们一些奖励、意义、目的感或与他人的联系感等方面"。保护性因素能降低自杀意念和自杀行为风险，在风险评估和支持性护理计划中都发挥着重要作用。

The NZGG (2003) define protective factors as "aspects of a person's life that give them some reward, meaning or sense of purpose, or sense of connection with others". Protective factors are associated with a decreased risk for suicide ideation and behaviour and therefore play a major part in both risk assessment and supportive care planning.

与保护作用相关的因素可能包括内部力量，如患者自身的应对技巧和自信，以及外部力量，如社会支持系统和精神卫生资源渠道（Holkup，2002）。此外，积极的治疗性关系也被认为对自杀行为有保护作用（APA，2003；NZGG，2003）。

Factors associated with protective effects may include internal strengths, such as the client's own coping skills and self-confidence, as well as external strengths, such as social support systems and access to mental health resources. Moreover, a positive therapeutic relationship has also been suggested to be protective against suicide behaviours.

保护性因素可以通过临床访谈来评估。通过询问个体是什么原因使他/她到目前为止没有执行这个计划，由此得出保护因素（Holkup，2002）。

Protective factors may be assessed through clinical interviews. It has been suggested that through asking the person what has kept him/her from acting out the plan thus far, you may illuminate protective factors.

不自杀合同

No-Suicide Contracts

文献表明，尽管缺乏实证证据来支持不自杀合同使用，医疗保健专业人员经常使用它作为评估和管理工具（APA，2003；Farrow，2002）。不自杀合同不能保证个体的安全，因此不应将其作为个体是否试图结束生命的唯一指标（Farrow，2003；NZGG，2003）。

The literature suggests that no-suicide contracts are frequently employed as assessment and management tools by health care professionals despite the lack of empirical evidence to support their use. No-suicide contracts do not guarantee a person's safety, thus should not be relied upon as the sole indicator as to whether a person may try to end his or her life.

虽然没有标准的定义,但不自杀合同实质上是指患者与临床医生之间关于患者不会自杀的口头或书面协议。在文献中,不自杀合同也可以被称为不自杀预防合同、不伤害合同、不自杀决定、安全协议、安全合同、自杀协议和继续生存契约(APA, 2003; Farrow, 2002; Rudd, Mandrusiak and Joiner, 2006)。

Although there is no standard definition, a no-suicide contract essentially refers to a verbal or written agreement between a patient and a clinician that the patient will not kill themselves. Within the literature, no-suicide contracts may also be referred to as no-suicide prevention contracts, no-harm contracts, no-suicide decisions, safety agreements, contracts, suicide agreements and contracting to stay alive.

不自杀合同的共同组成部分包括明确声明不自杀或伤害自己、协议期限的细节以及患者无法遵守条件的应急计划(Centre for Suicide Prevention, 2002b; Rudd et al., 2006)。应谨慎使用不自杀合同,它不适用于曾有过自杀未遂、情绪激动、焦虑、精神病、冲动或中毒的患者(APA, 2003; Murray and Hauenstein, 2008)。

Common components of a no-suicide contract include an explicit statement not to kill or harm oneself, details about duration of the agreement and contingency plans should the client be unable to keep the conditions. If used, no-suicide contracts should be used with caution, and not used with clients who have had previous suicide attempts, being agitated, psychotic, and impulsive or intoxicated.

尽管一致认为不应在治疗性关系中使用不自杀合同,但文献表明护士在紧急或社区危机情况中经常使用这种工具(Farrow, 2003)。因此,不自杀合同可能会提供一种虚假的安全感,仅仅是缓解医疗专业人员的焦虑感。

Despite the consensus that no-suicide contracts should only be used within the context of a therapeutic relationship, the literature suggests that nurses often utilize such tools in emergency or community crisis situations. As a result, the no-suicide contract may provide a false sense of security and little more than alleviation of anxiety on the part of the health care professional.

尽管缺乏实证证据来支持它的使用,专家组建议,使用不自杀合同应谨慎,并且只能在治疗关系下和更全面的评估和管理计划的前提下使用。如果决定将不自杀合同作为治疗计划的一部分,则不应单独进行,而应在多学科小组包括患者参与的范围内进行。

Despite the lack of empirical evidence to support their use, the panel suggests that if used, no-suicide contracts be used with caution and only within the context of a therapeutic relationship and a more comprehensive assessment and management plan. If, and when, a decision is made to include a no-suicide contract as part of the treatment plan, it should not be done in isolation, but rather within the context of the multidisciplinary team, inclusive of the client.

虽然不自杀合同可以作为一种授权手段使患者参与制定治疗计划,当事人是否愿意订立这样的协议,不应作为一个绝对表明他/她是否会继续伤害自己或自杀的指标(APA, 2003)。如果患者不愿意签订不自杀合同,这可能表明他/她对于遵守合同的矛盾心理和没有能力遵守合同,需要进一步评估和探讨其他管理办法。

Although no-suicide contracts can be used as a means to empower the client by involving him/her in the development of his/her treatment plan, the client's willingness to enter into such an agreement should not be used as an absolute indicator as to whether he/she may go on to harm or kill oneself. Should a client be unwilling to enter into a no-suicide contract, this may be indicative of ambivalence and his/her inability to adhere to the contract, necessitating further assessment and exploration of other management options.

相反,患者愿意将不自杀合同作为其管理计划的一部分,并不能保证他/她不会继续自我伤害或自杀。在Kroll(2007)的一项研究中,152名精神科医生使用不自杀合同,41%的人报告称,他们有病人在达成协议后自杀未遂或自杀死亡。需要进行更多的研究,以确定不自杀合同的效力。

On the contrary, a client's willingness to include a no-suicide contract as part of their management plan does not guarantee that he or she will not go on to harm or kill oneself. In a study by Kroll (2007), of the 152 psychiatrists who used no-suicide contracts, 41% reported that they had patients who attempted or killed oneself after entering into such an agreement. Additional research is required to determine the efficacy of the no-suicide contract.

建议6c:护士应从所有现有来源获得间接信息——家庭、朋友、社区支持、医疗记录和精神卫生专业人员。(Ⅳ类证据)

Recommendation 6c: The nurse should obtain collateral information from all available sources—family, friends, community supports, medical records and mental health professionals. (Type Ⅳ Evidence)

这些信息可以提供关于患者的精神状态或行为的重要信息,这些信息可能暗示着自杀意念,以及最近可能对患者产生影响的任何压力源(APA,2003; NZGG,2003)。护士必须考虑保密问题,并了解有关的隐私法例。在获得间接信息之前,必须征得患者的同意。

Such information can provide important information about the client's mental state or behaviour that may indicate suicidal ideation, as well as any recent stressors that may be impacting on the client. It is important for the nurse to consider the issue of confidentiality and understand the relevant privacy legislation. The client's consent for obtaining collateral information must be sought prior to doing so.

如果患者不希望与家人或其他重要的人联系,而这又不危害患者的安全,则必须保密(NZGG,2003)。然而,在紧急情况下,为了维护患者或其他人的安全,允许护士未经同意获得间接信息(APA,2003;Cavoukian,2004;NZGG, 2003)。

If the client does not want his/her family members or significant others to be contacted and this does not compromise the safety of the client, then confidentiality must be maintained. However, in emergency situations, it is permissible to obtain collateral information without consent in order to maintain the safety of the client or others.

重要的是,当与家庭成员或其他重要的人交流以获取间接信息时,必须理解这种交流的目的是获取信息,而不是提供信息。在无法获得间接信息的潜在来源或所获得的信息中存在不一致的情况下,可能会出现困难。在这些情况下,可能需要进行进一步的调查,以帮助护士和卫生保健小组加深对特定临床情景的理解。

Importantly, when interacting with family members or significant others to obtain collateral information, it must be understood that the goal of such communication is to acquire information, not to provide information. Challenges may arise in cases where potential sources of collateral information are not available or there are inconsistencies in the information received. In these situations, further investigation may be warranted to help the nurse and health care team develop an understanding of the particular clinical scenario.

建议7:护士应确保观察和治疗的投入能反映患者自杀风险的变化。(Ⅳ类证据)

Recommendation 7: The nurse should ensure that observation and therapeutic engagement reflects the client's changing suicide risk. (Type Ⅳ Evidence)

对有自杀风险的人立即进行观察。一旦完成全面评估,应根据需要调整支持和观察等级。在国际文献(Jones *et al.*,2000;O'Brien and Cole,2003;

Reynolds *et al.*，2005)和指南(CRAG，2002；NZGG，2003)中，观察实践有很大的差异，特别是关于不同观察级别的特征以及可以启动或改变观测等级的条件。

Observation begins immediately for anyone identified as a suicide risk. Once a comprehensive assessment is completed, the level of support and observation should be adapted as required. There is much variation in observation practices among international literature and guidelines, particularly relating to the attributes of different levels of observation and the conditions by which observation levels can be initiated or changed.

因此，观察的目的是向缺乏防止自杀意念能力的患者提供支持，本指南建议，监测等级应反映患者风险水平的变化，这取决于临床判断和与卫生保健小组的协作(Clinical Resource and Audit Group，2002；NZGG，2003)。患者对理解和控制自伤行为的信心是决定最合适的观察等级的一个重要因素(Murray and Hauenstein，2008)。

Whereby the purpose of observation is to provide support to clients who lack the capacity to prevent acting on suicide ideation, this guideline recommends that the level of monitoring reflect the client's changing level of risk, as determined by clinical judgment and collaboration with the health care team. The client's confidence in understanding and controlling self-harm behaviour is an important factor for determining the most appropriate observation level.

观察等级的决策还应考虑自杀风险等级、现有的监测支持、观察者提供的技能水平、环境的适宜性和组织政策(Clinical Resource and Audit Group，2002)。在医院或组织环境中，这包括随时了解患者的行踪，以及使患者始终在视线和接触范围内(CRAG，2002)。

Decision-making regarding observation levels should also involve a consideration of the level of suicide risk, existing support for monitoring, the skill level of the individuals providing observation, the suitability of the environment and organizational policies. In hospital or organizational settings, this may range from knowledge of the clients' whereabouts at all times, to the client being constantly in sight and within arm's reach.

虽然观察应由受过专业知识和技能培训的人进行，但非专业人员(如家庭成员)的作用是可适当讨论和考虑的(CRAG，2002)。

Although observation should be carried by individuals trained with the appropriate knowledge and skills, the role of the non-professional (e.g., family members) is one for local discussion and consideration.

重要的是,清晰的记录有助于团队内部的沟通,并有助于对观察需求的持续评估(CRAG,2002)。患者和其他重要的人也应该被告知有关观察的决定(CRAG,2002),并酌情纳入决策。

Importantly, clear documentation facilitates communication within the team and the ongoing assessment of the need for observation. The client and significant others should also be informed about the decisions made regarding observation and included in decision-making as appropriate.

建议 8:护士应与患者协作,理解患者的观点和满足患者的需求。(Ⅳ类证据)

Recommendation 8: The nurse should work collaboratively with the client to understand his/her perspective and meet his/her needs. (Type Ⅳ Evidence)

自杀者更有可能意识到他们有需求,并且许多人认为他们的需求没有得到充分满足。(Pirkis *et al*., 2001)。为了满足患者的需要,护士应该运用有效的沟通技巧,例如倾听和肯定,以便于患者能够从他们自己的角度来表达他们的故事和需求(Gough, 2005; Murray and Hauenstein, 2008; O'Brien and Cole, 2003)。

Suicide persons are more likely to perceive they have needs, and many believe their needs have not been fully met. To assist in meeting the needs of the client, the nurse should utilize effective communication techniques, such as listening and validating, so that the client is able to convey his/her story and needs from their own perspective.

Cdereke and Ojehagen (2002) 评估了患者在五个一般方面的需求(基本需求、健康需求、社会需求、日常功能的需求、服务的需求),发现在自杀未遂后的前12个月中,基本需求、社会需求和医疗保健需求在未得到满足的需求中排名最高。

Cdereke and Ojehagen (2002) assessed the needs of clients in five general areas (basic, health aspects, social needs, daily functioning and services), and found that basic needs, social needs and health-care needs ranked the highest as being unmet during the first 12 months post-suicide attempt.

马斯洛层次理论(Maslow, 1943)提供了相关需求的框架,如图 1.1 所示,其中指出要先满足低层次需求,如食物、住宿,然后是更高层次的需求,如自我价值感。采用以患者为中心和有文化能力的方法去评估,可以确定个人的具体需求。

Maslow's Hierarchy of Needs offers a framework for the consideration of needs, as shown in Figure 1.1, where lower-level needs, such as food and shelter, must be met before higher-level needs, such as a sense of self-worth. Using a client-centred and culturally competent approach to assessment, the specific needs of the individual can be identified.

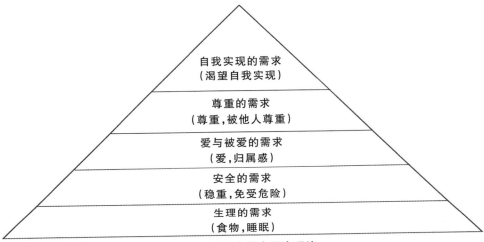

图1.1 马斯洛需求层次理论

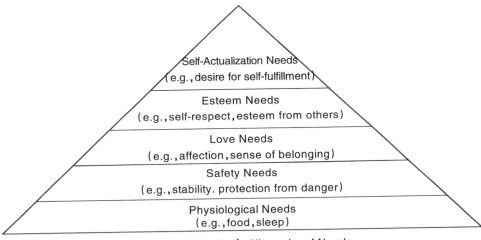

Figure 1.1 Maslow's Hierarchy of Needs

在确定自杀高风险患者的需求后,护士应当积极参与患者的治疗,制定策略来满足患者这些需求。这些策略可能包括以下几个方面:

Following the identification of needs, the nurse should be actively involved with the client to develop strategies to meet these needs. Such strategies may involve the following:

• 获得服务的便利途径(Eagles *et al.*, 2003);

• 咨询服务、药物治疗、提供信息(Pirkis *et al.*, 2001);

• 积极与外界联系；

• 适当地鼓励患者积极融入社会环境,强化患者的自我意识,改变厌恶的人际关系交往模式(O'Brien and Cole, 2003)；

• 通过协作和团队合作来确保一致的护理方法。

• Facilitating access to services；

• Counseling, medication and information；

• Active outreach；

• Encouragement of active participation in social environments, as appropriate, to strengthen the client's ego and modify aversive interpersonal patterns；

• Using collaboration and teamwork to ensure a consistent approach to care.

协作是为了实现共同的目标而相互分享和共同工作,从而使所有的人或群体都得到认可和促进成长。(Stanhope and Lancaster, 2000)。

Collaboration is the mutual sharing and working together in order to achieve common goals in such a way that all persons or groups are recognized and growth is enhanced.

实践框

Practice Box

加强患者自我价值感的可能性策略

Possible Strategies for Affirming a Client's Self-Worth

(RNAO Development Panel, 2008)

肯定、尊重、共情很大程度上证明你认可一个人的价值。以下是一些与患者分享的其他人发现自我价值的方法。

Validation, respect and compassion go a long way to demonstrate that you recognize the person's worth. Here are some ways to share with the client that other people see their worth：

■鼓励患者善待并理解自己。支持他们通过写日记记录他们的想法,重新积极地思考他们任何消极的想法。

■和患者对话时，认可他们的优势。

■与患者合作，制定可实现的日常目标并完成这些目标。

■帮助患者设想改变。帮助患者描述他们渴望被改变的行为。

■帮助患者制定对小成就的奖励。

■在事情不尽如人意时，开导患者不要自责。

■帮助患者用积极的想法对抗消极的想法。

■Encourage the client to be kind and understanding with themselves. Support the use of a diary to journal their thoughts and to positively reframe any negative thoughts.

■When dialoguing with the client, acknowledge their strengths.

■ Work with client to set achievable daily goals and to accomplish them.

■ Help the client to visualize change. Help the client describe the desired changed behaviour.

■ Help the client establish rewards for small accomplishments.

■ Help the client not to blame themselves when something does not go as they wanted.

■ Assist the client to counteract negative thoughts with positive thoughts.

IV 类证据

Type IV Evidence

建议 9:护士应运用护患共同解决问题的方法,来促进患者理解如何看待自己的问题和形成解决办法。(IV 类证据)

Recommendation 9: The nurse should use a mutual problem-solving (client-nurse) approach to facilitate the client's understanding of how they perceive their own problems and generate solutions. (Type IV Evidence)

自杀意念和自杀行为常常是人们应对某种个人无法承受的情况时的一种表现,它与心理和情感上的痛苦有关(Berlim *et al.*, 2003)。因此,自杀并不一定表达对死亡的渴望,当提供患者其他可选择的应对策略进行干预时,可以预防自杀。根据 Sakinofsky(2007b)的说法,降低自杀风险包括防止患者因问题累积而陷入不堪重负的困境。

Suicide ideation and behaviour often represent a way of coping with situations that the individual perceives to be unbearable and can be linked to psychological and emotional pain. As such, suicidality does not necessarily communicate a desire to die and can be influenced by interventions which provide the individual with alternative coping strategies. According to Sakinofsky (2007b), reducing suicide risk involves preventing the client from being overwhelmed by the predicament caused by an accumulation of problems.

很多患者可能不太理解,他们的压力源和他们自杀意念或者自杀行为之间的联系(Murray and Hauenstein, 2008)。通过帮助患者认识如何看待自己的问题,并提出解决这些问题(即自杀)的方法,护士可以帮助患者了解是什么导致了他们的自杀倾向,在未来如何采用多种选择解决问题(Fontaine, 2003; Murray and Hauenstein, 2008)。

Many clients may not understand the connection between their stressors and their suicide thoughts or behaviour. By assisting individuals to recognize how they perceive their problems and generate solutions to these problems (i.e., suicide), the nurse can facilitate the client's understanding of what has led to their suicidality, and how to use a variety of options in solving future problems.

鼓励患者参与制定他们自己的策略,不仅能确保这些策略的适当性,还能帮助患者重新获得对当下情形的控制感。对患者和其家人而言，最重要的过程是如何解决问题(Fontaine，2003)。在运用问题解决方法时，根据患者的意愿和患者处于自主或者依赖的不同情形来调整解决方法也很重要。自主型患者陷入困境时需要借助他人的支持；而依赖型患者需要感觉不被抛弃(Burgess，1998)。

Promoting the client's involvement in generating their own strategies not only ensures the appropriateness of such strategies, but also helps the client regain a sense of control regarding the situation. The most important process for clients and families is how to solve problems. When applying a problem-solving approach, it is also important to tailor this approach basing on the client's readiness and where the client is on the autonomous or dependent continuum. Autonomous clients feel trapped and need support; dependent clients need to feel unabandoned.

尽管问题解决方法在心理健康护理实践中被广泛使用，但是缺乏围绕问题解决方法的本质属性与有效的经验知识体系。然而，尽管在证据基础上存在差距，问题解决方法在降低反复蓄意自伤事件方面已经有所成效(Hawton *et al.*，2006；Mustafa Soomro，2006)，并和冲动诱因的管理有关(Fontaine，2003)。

Although it is widely used in mental health nursing practice, the body of empirical knowledge surrounding the essential attributes and effectiveness of the problem-solving approach is lacking. However, despite the gaps in the evidence base, problem-solving therapy has shown promise in reducing repeated episodes of deliberate self-harm and has been linked to the management of triggers to impulsivity.

一些处于危机中的患者可能会有思维不清晰、思维混乱和解决问题的困难。要了解如何与这类患者合作，尤其是关于探索患者应对和商定行动计划方面，请参阅RNAO最佳实践指南危机干预(RNAO，2006b)。

Some clients in crisis may have difficulty thinking clearly, be confused and have difficulty solving problems. For understanding of how to work with such clients, especially in regard to exploring client-coping and negotiating an action plan, please refer to the RNAO Best Practice Guideline Crisis Intervention.

进一步的研究集中在将问题解决疗法作为一种护理干预措施。Taylor(2000)指出，安全和专业的护理依赖于良好的临床问题解决能力。问题解决的定义是"对关注的问题提出可能的解决方案，并应成为所有专业人员实践中的一个固有部分"(Eisenhauer and Gendrop，1990，as cited in Taylor，2000)。

Further research focused on problem-solving therapy as a nursing intervention. Taylor (2000) stated that the ability of the nurse to provide safe, competent care depended on good clinical problem-solving skills. Problem-solving is defined as "the generation of possible solutions to an issue of concern, and therefore needs to be an inherent part of the practice of all professionals".

这个过程开始于护士确诊患者问题的时刻,持续到做出将减轻或者解决问题的决定,如图1.2所示。对问题解决途径的一个建议性框架将在下一页提供。

This process begins when a client problem is identified by a nurse and persists through to the point where a decision is made that will alleviate or solve the problem, as shown in Figure 1.2. A suggested framework for a problem-solving approach is as follows.

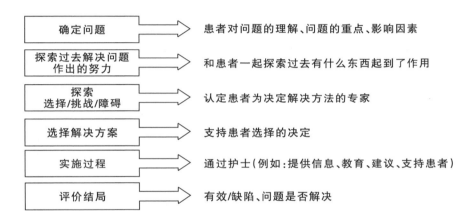

图1.2 问题解决方法途径

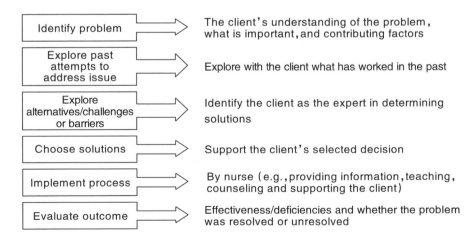

Figure 1.2 Problem-Solving Approach to Solution

实践框

Practice Box

使用问题解决方法的实践策略

Practice Strategies Using a Problem-Solving Approach to Solutions

（RNAO Development Panel, 2008）

A. 确定问题

①让患者描述正在发生的事情。还有哪些人参与其中？

②帮助患者分解问题，把重点放在当前问题（优先事项）。

③可能的自毁行为的诱发因素和模式是什么？

④通过使用日记来回忆和详细描述关系、情绪、诱因、自伤行为模式，帮助患者进行自我审视。

A. Identify Problem

①Ask the client to describe what is happening. Who are the other people involved?

②Help the client break down the problem to focus on the immediate issue （priority）.

③What are the triggers and patterns of possible self-destructive acts?

④Assist the client to self-monitor through the use of diaries to recall and detail relationships, moods, triggers, and patterns of self-harm behaviour.

B. 探索过去解决问题做出的努力

①帮助患者确定过去哪些工作是有效的。

②帮助患者确定支持/资源/个人优势。

B. Explore Past Attempts to Address Issue

①Help the client identify what has worked in the past.

②Help the client identify support/resources/personal strengths.

C. 探索替代方案/挑战以确定解决方案

①确定提供改变和一些控制的小步骤。

②检查药物在减轻焦虑方面的作用（APA, 2003）。

③探索安全的选择，例如呼吸和放松（Frazier *et al.*, 2003）。

C. Explore Alternatives/Challenges or barriers

①Identify small steps that will provide change and some control.

②Examine the role of medications to reduce anxiety.

③Explore safe alternatives, such as breathing and relaxation.

D. 选择解决方案

重点在于帮助患者确定小步骤、应对策略、减轻压力、解决问题、对结果的自我反省。

D. Choose Solutions

Focus on helping the client identify small steps, coping strategies, stress reduction, problem-solving and self-examination of results.

E. 实施过程

①确定患者何时会"停下来思考"并采取一致同意的行动。

②记录成功、情感和学习是有帮助的（Fontaine, 2003）。

③提供具有时间限制的治疗疗程，帮助患者解决目前的人际关系问题（Gaynes *et al*.，2004）。

E. Implement Process

①Identify when the patient will "stop and think" and use collaboratively agreed upon action.

②Journaling successes, emotions, and learning is helpful.

③Provide time-limited therapeutic sessions to assist the client in resolving current interpersonal problems.

F. 评价结果

①通过与患者讨论他们的能力和局限性，促进他们进行真实的自我评价。帮助患者反映目标明确的任务结果。

②鼓励——指出小成功，提高患者自我评价的能力（Fontaine，2003）。

F. Evaluate Outcomes

①Promote realistic self-appraisal through discussing with the client their abilities and limitations. Help the client reflect outcomes of purposeful tasks.

②Encourage—point out small successes and reinforce the client's ability to appraise themselves.

Ⅳ类证据

Type Ⅳ Evidence

建议10：护士应培养自杀患者的希望。（Ⅳ类证据）

Recommendation 10：The nurse should foster hope with the suicide client. (Type Ⅳ Evidence)

众所周知,绝望与自杀、自杀未遂的风险以及自杀意念强度的增加有关(APA，2003)。绝望是一种对自己的生活状况或境遇的改变或改善不抱希望的感觉,其特征是感觉力不胜任和无力为自己采取行动。(Murray and Hauenstein，2008)。

It is well established that hopelessness is associated with an increased risk for suicide and suicide attempts, and the increased level of suicide intent. Hopelessness, characterized by feelings of inadequacy and an inability to act on one's own behalf, is a perception of having no hope that one's life situation or circumstance will change or improve.

希望的想法在痊愈的背景下也处于有利地位。当患者感到绝望时,护士可以灌输或培养患者对未来的希望感(MacLeod *et al*.，1997)。希望和关怀之间有着密切的关系(Cutcliffe and Barker，2002)。通过与患者建立治疗性关系,护士传达包容和接纳。患者如何感受自己的境遇,极大地影响着他如何看待自己。

The idea of hope is also well situated in the context of recovery. When the client is experiencing hopelessness, the nurse can instill or foster a sense of hope for the future. There is a strong relationship between hope and caring. By forming a therapeutic relationship with the client, the nurse conveys tolerance and acceptance. How a client perceives they are treated significantly impacts how the client feels about themselves.

自杀患者经常感到一种无可抗拒的绝望感,并且可能会把它投射到护士身上。护士必须意识到他/她自己的希望感和无望感,以便能够支持病人。为了使护士的绝望感或负罪感不被传达给患者,对患者感到绝望的护士需要通过小组会议或临床监督来解决问题。

Suicide clients often feel an overpowering sense of hopelessness and may project that to the nurse. The nurse must be aware of his/her own feelings of hopefulness and hopelessness in order to be able to support the client. The nurse who is feeling hopeless about the client needs to address this through either a team meeting or through clinical supervision, in order that the nurse's feelings of hopelessness or guilt are not conveyed to the client.

建议11:护士应了解目前的治疗方法,以便酌情提供宣传、转介、观察和健康教育干预措施。(Ⅳ类证据)

Recommendation 11: The nurse should be aware of current treatments in order to provide advocacy, referral, monitoring and health teaching interventions, as appropriate. (Type Ⅳ Evidence)

可用于管理患者自杀意念和自杀行为风险的治疗方式,包括心理疗法、精神药理学、电休克疗法(ECT)和补充或替代疗法(APA, 2003; Hawton et al., 2006; NZGG, 2003)。作为多学科团队的一部分,护士必须了解这些方式,以便酌情提供以患者为中心的宣传、观察和健康教育干预措施。

Treatment modalities that may be used to manage clients' risk for suicidal ideation and behaviour include: psychotherapy, psychopharmacology, electroconvulsive therapy (ECT) and complementary or alternative therapies. As part of the multidisciplinary team, the nurse must have knowledge of these modalities in order to provide client-centred interventions regarding advocacy, monitoring and health teaching, as appropriate.

这个领域提供了很多可以转介给专业技能人员(即注册护士、注册精神病学护士、高级实践护士、精神病医生和其他相关卫生专业人员)的机会。为了与以患者为中心和文化安全方法保持一致,探讨患者对各种治疗方案的认识和意义也很重要。

This area offers many opportunities for referral to persons who have specialized skills (i. e., RNs, RPNs, advanced practice nurses, psychiatrists and other allied health professionals). In keeping with the client-centred and culturally safe approach, it is also important to explore the client's knowledge and meaning of various treatment options.

心理疗法

Psychotherapy

大多关于心理治疗方式的研究,如认知行为疗法、辩证行为疗法,侧重其在处理与特定疾病相关的心理症状和危险因素的应用上(APA, 2003),例如边缘型人格障碍(Linehan, 1993)和精神分裂症(Mamo, 2007)。

Most studies regarding psychotherapeutic modalities, such as Cognitive Behavioural Therapy and Dialectical Behavioural Therapy, are focused on its use in addressing psychosocial symptoms and risk factors related to specific disorders, such as borderline personality disorder and schizophrenia.

其他指南和系统评价指出,缺乏严谨的研究来直接评估这些方式在降低自杀率方面的有效性(APA, 2003; Hawton *et al.*, 2006; Mann *et al.*, 2005; Mustafa Soomro, 2006)。然而,尽管文献中存在空白,临床共识仍然表明,心理社会干预和特定的心理治疗方法对自杀患者是有益的(APA, 2003)。

Other guidelines and systematic reviews note the paucity of rigorous studies that directly evaluate the effectiveness of these modalities on reducing suicidality. However, despite gaps in the literature, clinical consensus continues to suggest that psychosocial interventions and specific psychotherapeutic approaches are of benefit to the suicide client.

心理疗法是"心理健康专家与患者讨论问题和感受,以此找到解决办法的一种心理疾病治疗方法。心理疗法可以帮助个人改变他们的思维和行为模式,或者理解过去的经历如何影响当前的行为"(国家心理健康词汇研究所,2005)。

Psychotherapy is a "treatment method for mental illness in which a mental health professional and a patient discuss problems and feelings to find solutions. Psychotherapy can help individuals change their thinking and behaviour patterns or understanding how past experience affects current behaviour".

精神药理学

Psychopharmacology

精神药理学是药理学的一个分支学科,包括影响大脑和精神疾病相关行为的药物使用(Austin and Boyd, 2008)。治疗抑郁和焦虑的药物在对有自杀意念和行为风险患者的照护中也发挥着作用(APA, 2003; Diaconu and Turecki, 2007; Sher, Oquendo and Mann, 2001)。护士应具备知识和技能来宣传、监测、支持并向病人和家属提供有关使用精神药理学作为潜在治疗方式的健康教育。

Psychopharmacology is a subspecialty of pharmacology that includes medications used to affect the brain and behaviours related to psychiatric disorders. Medications in treatment of depression and anxiety may also play a role in caring for clients at risk for suicide ideation and behaviour. The nurse should possess the knowledge and skills to advocate for, monitor, support and provide health teaching to the client and family related to the use of psychopharmacology as a potential treatment modality.

虽然药物有助于控制与自杀风险有关的症状,但它们的使用不一定构成保护因素(Baldessarini *et al.*, 2005),因此,临床密切观察自杀患者精神药物的使用是很有必要的。观察患者服药需要了解患者的基线症状,以便这些症状可以与药物不良反应相关的症状进行比较(Baldessarini *et al.*, 2005; NZGG, 2003)。

Although medications may help to control symptoms related to suicide risk, their use does not necessarily constitute a protective factor and therefore, close clinical monitoring of psychopharmacology use with suicide clients is essential. Monitoring a client who is taking medications involves knowing the individual's baseline symptoms so that these symptoms can be compared with symptoms associated with adverse drug effects.

改良电休克疗法

Modified electroconvulsive therapy

改良电休克治疗(MECT),又称为无抽搐电休克疗法,是在通电治疗前,先注射适量的肌肉松弛剂,然后利用一定量的电流刺激大脑,引起患者意识丧失,从而达到无抽搐发作而治疗精神病的一种方法。其可改善ECT治疗相关弊端,如在治疗前对患者进行全身麻醉、肌肉松弛等处理,大大降低了患者发生肌肉强收缩的可能性。美国精神病学会(American Psychiatric Association, APA)指出,ECT是治疗精神疾病或自杀的最佳方法。长期以来,ECT主要被用于治疗情感障碍患者自杀行为,被推荐为治疗高自杀风险的重要措施。由于没有证据显示在紧急电休克治疗后,自杀风险会长期或持续降低,在随后的数周和数月内,通常需要密切观察和使用精神药物做辅助治疗。

Modified electroconvulsive therapy(MECT), also known as convulsion-free electroconvulsive therapy, is a method of treating psychosis without convulsive seizures by injecting an appropriate amount of muscle relaxant and then stimulating the brain with a certain amount of electric current before the electroconvulsive therapy. It can improve the drawbacks related to ECT treatment, such as general anesthesia and muscle relaxation before treatment, which greatly reduces the possibility of strong muscle contraction in patients. ECT is considered the best treatment for mental illness or suicide, according to the American Psychiatric Association (APA). For a long time, ECT has been mainly used for the treatment of suicide behavior in patients with mood disorders, and has been recommended as an important measure for the treatment of high suicide risk. Since there is no evidence of a long-term or sustained reduction in the risk of suicide following emergency electroconvulsive therapy, close observation and the use of psychotropic drugs as adjuvant therapy are often required in the following weeks and months.

补充和替代方式

Complementary and Alternative Modalities

补充和替代方式(CAM)被患者用作辅助治疗方式,来治疗与抑郁、焦虑或精神疾病有关的自杀行为(Brugha et al., 1998; Linde et al., 2001; Williams et al., 2000)。其治疗方式包括草药治疗、膳食补充、按摩/反射疗法、芳香疗法、针灸、瑜珈、冥想、灵气和音乐(Brugha et al., 2004; Weier and Beal, 2004)。

Complementary and alternative modalities (CAM) are used by clients as an adjunct treatment modality to manage their suicide behaviour related to depression, anxiety or a mental illness. These include treatment modalities, such as herbal remedies, dietary supplements, massages/reflexology, aromatherapy, acupuncture, yoga, meditation, reiki and music.

护士必须探讨患者对补充和替代方式的理解和使用,以确保患者的安全,特别是常规精神药物的额外使用,还需要考虑具体的文化模式。护士需要尊重族群内部和各民族文化群体之间的差异,而这些差异通常被那些群体认为是不可替代的。

It is important for the nurse to explore the client's understanding and use of CAM in order to ensure that the client's safety is maintained, particularly with the additional use of conventional psychopharmacology. Culture-specific modalities also need to be considered. The nurse needs to be respectful of differences within, and across ethno-cultural groups that are not considered by people within those groups to be "alternative".

相反，文化模式是健康和福祉不可或缺的组成部分，它可以与西方药物和方法一起使用，也可以单独使用或完全不使用。例如，汗蒸房、烟熏、草药和很多其他传统方法被原住民使用（Waldram，1997）。

Rather, they are integral to health and well-being and may be used alongside western medicines and approaches, alone or not at all. For example, the sweatlodge, smudging, medicinal plants and many other traditional approaches are used by First Nations.

实践框

Practice Box

对患者使用补充和替代方式（CAM）的有效方法

Helpful approaches with the client using complementary and alternative modalities （CAM）

（RNAO Development Panel，2008）

①确认患者使用或考虑使用补充和替代治疗作为主要或辅助治疗方式。

②无论患者的选择或喜好如何，愿意并且准备好与患者合作。

③了解补充和替代治疗的使用范围和使用原因。

④了解常规治疗和替代治疗的区别。

⑤利用人际沟通技巧和治疗性干预措施：

■探讨患者对传统和替代治疗的信念和看法；

■询问患者目前的药物治疗，包括病人已经使用、尝试过和/或正在使用的非处方药和替代疗法；

■探讨患者对补充和/或替代疗法的认知，选择它的理由，以及对已知或感知利益的期望；

■了解患者对副作用的认知；

■掌握口服避孕药、抗凝剂和降压药等伴随药物的使用信息；

■必要时观察有害的药物相互作用；

■根据代理协议来记录。

①Acknowledge that the client uses or considers using complementary and alternative treatments as a primary or adjunct treatment modality.

②Be willing and prepared to work with the client，regardless of the client's choices or preferences.

③Know the range of complementary and alternative treatments used and the reasons for usage.

④Know the difference between conventional treatment and alternative treatment.

⑤Utilize interpersonal communication skills and therapeutic interventions to：

■Explore the client's beliefs and views about conventional and alternative treatment；

■Ask the client about current medication including over-the-counter medication and alternative therapy the client has used，tried and/ or is using；

■Explore the client's knowledge of complementary and/or alternative treatments，the reason for choosing CAM，and expectations of benefits known or perceived；

■Explore the client's knowledge of side effects；

■Possess knowledge to provide information on the use of concomitant drugs such as oral contraceptives， anticoagulants and antihypertensive medications；

■Observe for harmful drug interactions as necessary；

■Document as per agency protocol.

Ⅳ类证据

Type Ⅳ Evidence

建议12：护士可根据组织方案，发起并参与其他医疗团队成员的汇报过程。（Ⅳ类证据）

Recommendation 12：The nurse may initiate and participate in a debriefing process with other health care team members as per organizational protocol. （Type Ⅳ Evidence）

事后干预适用于受自杀死亡影响从而产生创伤后遗症的人群。"它涉及为失去亲人的幸存者提供心理健康和公共健康服务"，包括与所有需要帮助的受影响者合作（Shneidman，1981，as cited in Brock，2003；Wilson and Clark，2005）。"在自杀预防领域，'幸存者'一词是用来形容因他人自杀而失去一个重要关系人的人，它并不是指那些自杀未遂而幸存下来的人"（Ball and White，2005）。

Postvention deals with the traumatic after-effects for persons affected by death due to suicide. "It involves offering mental health and public health services to the bereaved survivors" and includes working with all persons affected who are in need. "In the suicide prevention field, 'survivor' is a word used to describe someone who has lost a significant other to suicide. It does not refer to those who have made a suicide attempt and survived".

自杀事后干预的主要目的是，帮助因自杀而遭受损失的人来恢复情绪，同时防止他传染或模仿自杀行为（Dafoe and Monk，2005）。有抑郁症史或早期有自杀意念或自杀行为的青年，特别有可能受到传染效应的影响，有计划地给予朋友和他人支持，能有效地减少那些受自杀死亡影响的人的心理、身体和社会方面的困难（Dafoe and Monk，2005）。

The primary purpose of suicide postvention is to support the emotional recovery of persons affected by a loss due to suicide while preventing contagion or imitative suicidal behaviour. Youth who have a history of depression or previous suicide ideation or behaviour may be at particular risk of the contagion effect and a planned response to support friends and others can be effective in reducing psychological, physical and social difficulties in persons affected by death due to suicide.

在对文献的系统回顾中，Sakinofsky（2007a）发现自杀对失去另一半的人有独特的影响。虽然这种丧失之痛与其他形式复杂的丧亲之痛有许多共同之处，但它所带来的,尤其如创伤性悲伤、羞愧感、自责感以及悲恸者对人生意义的不断探求,使得这种悲伤与众不同——自杀死亡者的亲属和朋友更容易患上抑郁症、创伤后应激障碍(PTSD),家庭凝聚力有时也受到挑战(Sakinofsky, 2007a)。

In a systematic review of the literature, Sakinofsky (2007a) found unique effects for people who have lost a significant other due to suicide. Although the grief associated with this kind of loss has much in common with other forms of complicated bereavement, especially traumatic grief, feelings such as shame, self-recrimination, and a perpetual search for meaning render it somewhat different—relatives and friends of persons who have died due to suicide are vulnerable to depressive illness and post-traumatic stress disorder (PTSD), and family cohesion is sometimes challenged.

关于自杀死亡后干预措施(事后干预)效果的研究相对较少,包含相关分析的荟萃分析"结论混杂,效应值可忽略不计"(Sakinofsky, 2007a)。护士与丧亲者合作的程度是可变的,受很多因素影响,如治疗机构的政策、丧亲者的偏好以及护士在治疗过程中的职业水准。

There are relatively few studies of the efficacy of interventions (postventions) following suicide deaths and meta-analyses of programs that allow this analysis are "mixed and show paltry effect sizes". The degree to which the nurse is involved in working with the bereaved person is variable and based on many factors, such as the policies of the practice setting, preferences of the bereaved individual and the level to which the nurse is competent to engage in the therapeutic relationship.

丧亲者可能会面临各种治疗机构,因此也可能是其他卫生专业人员来提供这些服务(如全科医生、法医、警察、宗教领袖和神职人员或专业丧亲顾问)。

Given the range of practice settings in which the bereaved may be encountered, it may be another health professional that may provide these services (i.e., general practitioners, coroners, police, religious leaders and the clergy or specialist bereavement counselors).

在提供事后干预支持时,重要的是对个人讨论死亡和丧亲的意愿保持敏感。建议临床医生应避免大肆渲染死亡、美化或诋毁自杀受害者,或提供关于自杀行为的过多细节(Gould and Kramer, as cited in Brock, 2003)。此外,临床医生不应该把自己的信仰,包括宗教信仰,强加给患者。

When providing postvention support, it is important to be sensitive to the individual's readiness to discuss the death and bereavement. It is suggested that clinicians should avoid sensationalizing the death, glorifying or vilifying the suicide victim, or provide excessive details about the suicide act. In addition, clinicians should not impose their own beliefs, including religious beliefs, onto the client.

现在许多学校、机构和社区的自杀事后干预服务,通常包括心理或危机事件汇报。汇报通常是在自杀事件发生后第一时间召开的一个单独会议。它的使用是基于这样的假设,即事后汇报将尽量减少创伤后应激障碍和其他对创伤情况的不良反应。尽管这种干预对参加者的好处尚不明确,但它的使用已经变得广泛起来。

Many school, institutional and community postvention services after suicide now routinely include psychological, or critical incident debriefing. This debriefing is commonly delivered as a single session in the immediate aftermath of the suicide. Its use is predicated upon the assumption that debriefing will minimize PTSD and other adverse reactions to traumatic situations. The use of this intervention has become extensive despite the fact that its benefits to participants have not been clearly established.

近期对心理汇报的随机对照试验的回顾表明,它不一定能有效地减轻创伤后应激障碍,减少精神病患病率,缓解抑郁症、焦虑或精神痛苦症状,实际上,它可能会增加创伤后应激障碍的风险。这一结论要求对这一领域的实践进行严格的审查,特别是要考虑重大事件汇报可能产生有害影响的程度。

Recent reviews of randomized controlled trials of psychological debriefing have suggested that it is not necessarily effective in reducing PTSD, psychiatric morbidity, depression, anxiety or symptoms of distress and may, in fact, increase risk of PTSD. This conclusion invites a critical review of practice in this area and, particularly, consideration of the extent to which critical incident debriefing may have harmful effects.

然而,现在公众普遍期望对所有创伤性事件提供事后汇报,并且这些事件的受害者提出这一过程是有帮助的。考虑到事后汇报受欢迎的程度,撤回这项服务可能会很困难(Beautrais, 2004)。这些服务可以由心理咨询师和其他精神卫生专业人员提供,或由在自杀后干预计划方面具有专业知识及经验的专家顾问提供。

However, there is now widespread public expectation that debriefing should be provided for all traumatic incidents, and the victims of such incidents report that they find the process helpful. Given this level of popularity, it might be difficult to withdraw this service. These services could be delivered by counselors and other mental health professionals, or by specialist consultants with expertise and experience in facilitating postvention programs after committed suicide.

建议 13:当工作中面临有自杀意念和行为风险的成人时,护士应通过临床督导寻求支持,认识到自杀对自身的情绪影响,并加强临床实践。(Ⅳ类证据)

Recommendation 13: The nurse should seek support through clinical supervision when working with adults at risk for suicide ideation and behaviour to become aware of the emotional impact to the nurse and enhance clinical practice. (Type Ⅳ Evidence)

临床督导是一个支持性的互动过程,可以协助护士提高他们的知识和专业能力,同时也提供了一个反思和支持的机会。对照护有自杀倾向患者的护士进行临床监督的重要性与文献一致(Carlen and Bengtsson, 2007; Cutcliffe and Barker, 2002; Linehan, 1993; NCCMH, 2004; NZGG, 2003; Royal Australian and New Zealand College of Psychiatrists Clinical Practice Guidelines Team for Deliberate Self-harm, 2004)。照护有自杀意念或自杀行为风险的患者对护士产生了很大的压力;临床督导是帮助护士反思并保持与患者的治疗性关系的一种方法(Cutcliffe and Barker, 2002)。

Clinical supervision is a supportive, interactive process that assists nurses in enhancing their knowledge and professional abilities while offering an opportunity for reflection and support. The importance of clinical supervision for the nurse working with suicide clients is consistent with the literature. Working with clients who are at risk for suicide ideation or behaviour can be stressful for the nurse; clinical supervision is one way to help the nurse reflect and maintain a therapeutic relationship with the client.

由于临床监督是护士与导师或其他高级临床医生进行人际交往的过程,在此过程中,护士会探索、检查和解决自身实践中的各种挑战,这也是一个不涉及惩罚或评判的反思学习和专业提升的机会。它为护士提供了一个安全地思考移情和反移情可能出现问题的机会。

Since clinical supervision is an interpersonal process in which nurses engage with mentors or another senior clinician to explore, examine and work through various challenges in their own practice, it is also an opportunity for reflective learning and professional growth that does not involve penalties or judgment. It provides an opportunity for the nurse to reflect safely on issues of transference and counter-transference that may arise.

临床督导还可以潜在地减轻这项困难工作对护士自身心理、情感和身体健康的负面影响(NZGG，2003)。考虑到在整个护理过程中与自杀患者合作，可能带来重大的个人和专业挑战，建议将临床督导作为不断实践的一部分来实施。

It can also potentially mitigate the negative effects of this difficult work on the nurse's own mental, emotional, and physical health. Given the significant personal and professional challenges that may arise out of working with suicide clients across the continuum of care, it is suggested that clinical supervision be implemented as an ongoing part of practice.

小品文

Vignette

情景：某位护士一直在照护玛丽亚，玛丽亚是一名曾多次自杀未遂的年轻女子。在她上次住院期间，她对药物反应良好，并同意出院后去接受心理咨询。最近，玛丽亚和她的男友分居了，停止服药，终止咨询，并过量服用了她母亲的安眠药。她回到了同一个病区，感到非常抑郁和绝望。

Scenario：The nurse has been working with Maria, a young woman who has had multiple suicide attempts. During her last hospitalization, she responded well to medication and agreed to go to counseling after discharge. Recently, Maria separated from her boyfriend, stopped taking her medication, quit counseling, and took an overdose of her mother's sleeping medication. She has returned to the same unit and is feeling quite depressed and hopeless.

这位护士之前很喜欢玛丽亚，因为玛丽亚让她想起了她的妹妹，而且她认为在玛丽亚上一次住院期间她们建立了一种积极且富有成效的关系。然而这次入院，当这位护士被分配照顾玛丽亚时，她对玛丽亚态度生硬，并且每当玛丽亚开始谈论她的感受时，护士都不想听。她的同事注意到她很烦躁，并在回避这位患者。

The nurse liked Maria, who reminded her of her sister, and felt they had a positive, productive relationship during Maria's last admission. This admission, however, when the nurse is assigned to care for Maria, she is quite abrupt with Maria and does not want to listen whenever Maria begins to talk about her feelings. Her colleague notices that she is irritable and avoiding this client.

护士反思：这位护士的同事向她提及了她似乎对这名患者感到心烦，并询问她相关情况。起初，护士否认这一点，说她"只是累了"。后来，在开车回家时，她开始思考这个问题，并意识到她的同事是对的。

Nurse's Reflection：The nurse's colleague mentions to her that she seems upset with this patient and asks her about it. At first the nurse denies this, stating that she is "just tired". Later, when driving home she begins to think more about this and realizes that her colleague is right.

她对这名患者感到生气，但不知道为什么；护士意识到有些不对劲，她需要一些帮助来解决这个问题。护士记得他们所在病区的护理医生围绕患者照护问题为其他同事提供了很多帮助，还为工作人员提供临床督导。她决定和护理医生谈谈关于她对这名患者作出反应的困难。

She is feeling angry with this patient but isn't sure why; something is wrong and the nurse realizes that she needs some help to figure this out. The nurse remembers that the nurse clinician for their unit has been helpful to other colleagues around patient care issues, and that he offers clinical supervision to staff. She decides to speak to the nurse clinician about her difficulty responding to this client.

护士反应：护士安排与护理医生见面。起初，她不愿意说实话，但护理医生让她感到舒服，提醒她他是来帮助她的。她开始谈论这位患者，包括这个女人让她想起她妹妹的事实。当她谈论她是如何"为这个女人浪费她的时间"时，她开始感到愤怒。护理医生帮助护士认识到，她对这个女人很生气有多种原因。

Nurse's Response: The nurse arranges to meet with the nurse clinician. At first she is hesitant to speak honestly, but the nurse clinician makes her feel comfortable and reminds her that he is there to help her. She begins to talk about this client, including the fact that the woman reminds her of her sister. She starts to feel angry when talking about how she is "wasting her time with this woman". The nurse clinician helps her to realize that she is angry with this woman for many reasons.

首先，因为在护士花费所有时间和精力照顾和治疗这位患者后，这个患者又试图自杀；其次，因为这位患者让护士想起了她的妹妹，妹妹总是向她寻求帮助，但从来没有听从她的劝告。护理医生理解护士的反应，但也帮助她了解患者的感觉。有了这种理解，护士开始更好地照护患者。她还安排在一周内与护理医生会面，继续讨论这位患者。

First, because she tried to kill herself again after all the time and energy that was spent on her care and treatment, and second, because she reminds the nurse of her sister, who is always asking her for help but never following through. The nurse clinician supports the nurse's reaction, but also helps her see how the client may be feeling. With this understanding, the nurse begins to work more productively again with this client. She also arranges to meet with the nurse clinician in a week to continue to discuss this client.

2 患者自杀风险评估

2 Patient Suicide Risk Assessment

2.1 自杀风险评估的指示

2.1 Indication for Suicide Risk Assessment

对风险的评估应始终在全面评估的背景下进行。

The assessment of risk should always take place within the context of a comprehensive exam.

普遍筛查:认识到住院患者群体存在心理困扰的风险,许多医疗保健系统已开始将常规筛查作为定期健康维护的一部分。像PHQ-9(该工具包括一个关于存在自杀意念的问题)这样的工具被广泛接受并应用于初级保健机构的患者。

Universal Screening: Recognizing the risk of psychological distress in the hospitalized population, many healthcare systems have begun routine screening as part of regular health maintenance. Instruments like the PHQ-9 (which includes a question regarding presence of suicidal ideation) are widely accepted and administered to patients in primary care settings.

精神疾病(精神障碍):某些精神疾病被认为是自杀的危险因素,其特点是大概率具有自杀意念(例如抑郁症)。在这些疾病的治疗中确定自杀意念,要求对自杀风险进行正式的全面评估和管理。

Mental Disorders (Psychiatric Disorders): Certain mental illnesses are considered to be risk factors for suicide and are characterized by a high rate of suicide ideation (e. g., depression). Identification of suicide ideation in the management of these illnesses should prompt formal comprehensive assessment and management of the risk for suicide.

医学状况(慢性疼痛):在许多情况下,慢性疼痛和身体不适与功能障碍和残疾有关,可能会增加自杀想法和自杀意念。精神共病在患有疼痛症状的个体中很常见。

Medical Conditions (Chronic pain): In many cases chronic pain and physical discomfort is associated with functional difficulties and disabilities that may increase suicide thoughts and ideation. Psychiatric comorbidity is common among individuals with a pain condition.

疼痛、抑郁和残疾是相辅相成的。共病性精神健康障碍可能是造成背部、颈部和关节疼痛的原因。频繁出现的头痛和"其他"慢性疼痛可能会带来额外的风险,这是精神疾病未捕获的心理过程继发的。

Pain, depression, and disability are known to be mutually reinforcing. Back, neck and joint pain can be accounted for by comorbid mental health disorders. There may be additional risk accompanying frequent headaches and "other" chronic pain that is secondary to psychosocial processes not captured by mental disorders.

医学状况(睡眠障碍):睡眠障碍在各种精神疾病和医学状况中普遍存在,并与之紧密相关。主观和客观睡眠障碍似乎都预示着自杀风险增加。不同设计、方法、自杀行为评估的多项调查都发现,失眠和睡眠质量差的症状是重要的自杀危险因素。噩梦在有自杀倾向和无自杀倾向的重度抑郁症患者中也更常见。

Medical Conditions (Sleep disorder): Sleep disturbance is prevalent in and strongly associated with a variety of psychiatric and medical conditions. Both subjective and objective sleep disturbances appear to predict elevated risk for suicide. Multiple investigations, diverse in design, methodology, and the assessment of suicide behaviors identify insomnia and poor sleep quality symptoms as significant suicide risk factors. Nightmares also appear more common among suicide versus nonsuicide individuals with major depression.

指示性筛查:根据人口统计学特征、其所面临的威胁、生理特征、身体特征或相关疾病或症状的发生情况,某些患者群体被认为具有特定健康状况的高风险。

Indicated Screening: Certain groups of patients are considered to be at elevated risk for specific health conditions by the nature of a demographic characteristic, exposure to a threat, biological characteristic, physical characteristic, or occurrence of a related illness or symptom.

例如,心肌梗塞患者有抑郁的风险,孕妇或产后妇女有抑郁的风险,因此,高危人群可能需要重点筛查。在这些高危人群中,任何阳性筛查都应进行重点评估。

For example, myocardial infarction patients are at risk for depression, women during pregnancy or in postpartum period are at risk for depression. As such, high-risk groups may be subject to focused screening. Any positive screen in these high-risk groups should be followed by a focused assessment.

临床评估：当患者向医疗服务提供者抱怨有关抑郁症状或自杀想法时，重点是评估自杀行为的性质、程度和其他特征或自杀行为的风险，从而制定目标治疗计划。

Clinical Assessment：When patients present to a health care provider with complaints regarding symptoms of depression or suicide thoughts, the focus is on conducting an evaluation to assess the nature, extent and other characteristics of suicide behavior or risk for suicide behavior with the goal of formulating a treatment plan.

从本质上讲，患者已经进行了自我筛查，并且进行了正式评估以建立对现存问题的诊断或其他临床方案。不管精神病学诊断如何，随后的治疗干预措施都将首先解决自杀的想法和行为。

In essence, the patient has self-screened for evaluation, and formal assessment is conducted to establish a diagnostic or other clinical formulation of the presenting problem. The therapeutic interventions that follow will first address the suicide thoughts and behaviors regardless of the psychiatric diagnosis.

2.2 患者自杀的影响因素

2.2 Influencing Factors of Suicide in Patients

危险和保护因素的存在作为风险评估的一部分，应在患者的病历中注明。虽然在统计上已将特定因素确定为危险因素，但卫生保健服务提供者必须认识到，尽管危险因素可能是累积的，但它们不是绝对的，没有加权值。

Presence of risk and protective factors should be noted in the patient's chart as part of the risk assessment. Although certain factors have been identified statistically as risk factors, health care service provider must be aware that risk factors are not absolute and carry no weighted value, though they may be cumulative.

自杀和自杀行为会导致严重的个人、社会和经济后果。尽管这些后果很严重，但从统计数据来看，自杀和自杀行为很少见，甚至在高危人群中也是如此。从统计学上看，自杀的小概率也使得我们无法仅凭单个或者多个危险因素进行预测。

Suicide and suicide behaviors cause severe personal, social, and economic consequences. Despite the severity of these consequences, suicide and suicide behaviors are statistically rare, even in populations at risk. The statistical rarity of suicide also makes it impossible to predict on the basis of risk factors either alone or in combination.

对于临床医务工作者来说，知道哪些特定因素（如重度抑郁症、绝望、物质使用)会增加患者的相对自杀风险,可能会影响治疗计划,包括确定治疗环境。与此同时,即使知道危险因素存在,也不能使临床医务工作者去预测患者是否会或者何时会自杀死亡。

For the clinical medical worker, knowing that a particular factor (e.g., major depressive disorder, hopelessness, substance use) increases a patient's relative risk for suicide may affect the treatment plan, including determination of a treatment setting. At the same time, knowledge of risk factors will not permit the clinical medical worker to predict when or if a specific patient will die by suicide.

但这也并不意味着临床医务工作者可以忽略这些危险因素,或者认为自杀的患者是不可治愈的。相反,临床医务工作者最初的目标应该是通过对危险和保护因素的全面评估来估计患者的风险,其首要和持续的目标应该是降低自杀风险。

This does not mean that the clinical medical worker should ignore risk factors or view suicidal patients as untreatable. On the contrary, an initial goal of the clinical medical worker should be to estimate the patient's risk through knowledgeable assessment of risk and protective factors, with a primary and ongoing goal of reducing suicide risk .

导致自杀风险的因素

自杀的警告信号	警告信号指观察中的个人在不久的将来从事自杀行为的可能性增加的信号。警告信号向临床医生提供了切实的证据,表明一个人在短期内处于自杀的风险较高;并且这有可能发生在没有危险因素的情况下
急性危险因素	急性(短暂的)和压力发作、疾病或生活事件,这些事件虽然通常不是由内部产生的,但可以锻炼并考验一个人的应对能力
慢性危险因素（已存在）	相对持久或稳定的因素,可能会增加一个人对自杀行为的敏感性,例如遗传和神经生物学因素、性别、性格、文化、社会经济背景和孤立水平
保护因素	增强抵御的能力、素质、环境和个人资源;驱使个人成长、稳定、健康和增加应对不同生活事件的能力

Factors Contributing to Risk for Suicide

Warning Signs for Suicide	Warning signs are those observations that signal an increase in the probability that the person intends to engage in suicide behavior in the immediate future . Warning signs present tangible evidence to the clinician that a person is at heightened risk for suicide in the short term, and may be experienced in the absence of risk factors

续表

Acute Risk Factors	Acute (of brief duration) and stressful episodes, illnesses, or life events, while not usually internally derived, these events can build upon and challenge a person's coping skills
Chronic Risk Factors (Pre-Existing)	Relatively enduring or stable factors may increase a person's susceptibility to suicide behaviors, such as genetic and neurobiological factors, gender, personality, culture, socio-economic background and level of isolation
Protective Factors	Capacities, qualities, environmental and personal resources can increase resilience and drive an individual toward growth, stability and health, increasing the ability to cope with different life events

自杀风险的不同层级

自杀风险	自杀风险指标	影响因素	基于风险水平的初步行动
高急性风险	•持续的自杀意念或想法 •有强烈的计划或行动意图 •不能控制冲动 •最近有自杀尝试或准备行为	•急性状态的精神障碍或严重精神症状 •急性事件 •保护因素不足	•保持对患者的直接观察控制 •限制获得致命手段 •立即转送至急诊/紧急护理机构住院
中度急性风险	•当前有自杀意念或想法 •没有实施行为的意图 •能够控制冲动 •最近没有自杀尝试行为或准备行为或排练行为	•警示信号或危险因素的存在 •保护因素有限	•向行为健康提供者咨询完整的评估和干预 •限制获得致命手段 •联系急诊医疗保健机构,以确定转诊
低急性风险	•最近有自杀意念或想法 •没有行动意图或计划 •能够控制冲动 •无规划或排练自杀行为 •无自杀尝试	•保护因素的存在 •危险因素有限	•考虑咨询行为健康以确定是否需要转介或治疗 •处理现存问题 •解决安全问题 •记录护理过程及采取行动的理由

Different Levels of Suicide Risk

Risk of Suicide Attempt	Indicators of Suicide Risk	Contributing Factors	Initial Action Based on Level of Risk
High Acute Risk	• Persistent suicide ideation or thoughts • Strong intention to act or plan • Not able to control impulse • Recent suicide attempt or preparatory behavior	• Acute state of mental disorder or acute psychiatric symptoms • Acute precipitating events • Inadequate protective factors	• Maintaining direct observational control of the patient. • Limiting access to lethal means • Immediate transfer with escort to urgent/ emergency care settings for hospitalization
Intermediate Acute Risk	• Current suicide ideation or thoughts • No intention to act • Able to control the impulse • No recent attempt or preparatory behavior or rehearsal of act	• Existence of warning signs or risk factors • Limited protective factors	• Referring to behavioral health providers for complete evaluation and interventions • Limiting access to lethal means • Contacting behavioral health providers to determine acuity of referral
Low Acute Risk	• Recent suicide ideation or thoughts • No intention to act or plan • Able to control the impulse • No planning or rehearsing a suicide act • No previous attempt	• Existence of protective factors • Limited risk factors	• Considering consultation with behavioral health services to determine referral or treatment • Treating present problems • Addressing safety issues • Documenting the care and the rationale for action

2.2.1 自杀的危险因素

2.2.1 Risk Factors for Suicide

自杀通常发生在危机中,很少在没有其他重要因素的情况下发生。自杀行为发生,通常需要一个诱因,一个促发性事件或触发因素,以及实现该自杀行为的能力(方法和途径)。意识到这些因素,就可以在危机的各个阶段采取干预措施降低风险。

Suicide usually occurs in a crisis and rarely happens in the absence of other important factors. For a suicide act to take place it usually requires a predisposition, a precipitating event or trigger, and the capability (methods and access to means) to carry it through. Being aware of these allows possible interventions to decrease the risk at various stages of the crisis.

危险因素有助于将高风险人群与低风险人群区分开。危险因素可能是可改变的,也可能是不可改变的。可改变的和不可改变的危险因素都可以为风险形成提供信息,可改变的危险因素也可能是干预的目标。危险因素评估的目标将根据临床情况和护理水平而有所不同。

Risk factors help distinguish a higher risk group from a lower risk group. Risk factors may be modifiable and non-modifiable. Both modifiable and non-modifiable risk factors inform risk formulation and modifiable risk factors may also be targets of intervention. The goal of risk factor assessment will vary depending on the clinical setting and level of care.

危险因素的存在可能增加自杀的风险,但是危险的敏锐度是通过警告信号的存在而进一步确定的。例如,并非所有失业者都有自杀的危险。

The presence of risk factors may increase risk for suicide, but the acuity of risk is further established by the presence of warning signs. For example, not all persons who are unemployed are at risk for suicide.

然而,如果一个失业的人对他的未来变得越来越绝望,可能是由于极度经济困难或无力支撑家庭,并开始表现为缺乏目的性(自尊水平下降),那么这个人可能存在高自杀风险。

However, if an unemployed person becomes increasingly hopeless about his or her future, possibly due to extreme financial difficulties or inability to support family, and begins to express purposelessness (decrease of self-esteem), then that person may be at a high risk for suicide.

很难确切地预测某个人是否真的会出现自杀尝试行为。但是,我们要知道,在多数情况下,自杀死亡的人在自杀之前就已经向他人传达了自杀的想法和感受以及他们自杀的意图,并且暗示他们错过了拯救生命的机会。

Predicting with certainty whether any given individual will actually attempt suicide is difficult, if not impossible. However, it is important to know that in many cases, people who die by suicide have communicated suicidal thoughts and feelings and their intent to kill themselves to someone prior to the suicidal act, and suggested missed opportunities for life-saving interventions.

我们可以认识到行为的变化和危机的存在,这些危机使人们处于高风险中,并可能导致自杀行为。与该人接触的朋友、家人、管理者和重要联系人都可以提供帮助。

It is possible to recognize changes in behavior and the existence of crises that place people at a high risk and may precipitate suicidal behavior. Friends, family members, commanders, and relatives who come into contact with the person can help.

了解危险因素有助于我们提供针对性干预,以防止涉及个体的潜在破坏性过程。然后可以采取措施降低风险。例如,创伤事件、慢性病和残疾、缺乏社会支持和极端损失(如财务、个人、社会)以及药物滥用等经历对于理解风险的来源很重要。

Knowledge of risk factors may help to target intervention that will prevent the potentially destructive process in which a person is involved. Action may then be taken to reduce the risks. For example, experiences such as history of traumatic events, chronic illness and disability, lack of social support and extreme loss (i.e., financial, personal, social), and substance abuse are important for understanding the origins of risk.

在没有警告信号的情况下,这些危险因素可能代表自杀的风险较小。集中干预以减轻这些压力,可以降低风险并避免发展成自杀行为的警告信号。

These risk factors in the absence of warning signs may represent a less immediate risk for suicide. Focusing intervention to mitigate these stressors can reduce the risk and avoid the progression into warning signs of suicide behavior.

一旦做出自杀死亡的决定,自杀者可能会反常地表现得不那么焦虑,看起来更稳定了,从而导致临床医务工作者低估了自杀风险。因此,最近被认为具有自杀高风险的人的痛苦明显下降,需要引起谨慎和重新评估风险。

Once the decision to die by suicide is made, the suicide person may paradoxically appear less agitated and more stable, leading clinicians to underestimate suicide risk. Therefore, a sudden apparent decrease in distress in an individual recently deemed to be at a high risk of suicide warrants caution and reassessment or risk.

可能增加风险的因素或可能降低风险的因素是那些被发现在统计学上与自杀行为相关或不相关的因素。它们不一定存在因果关系。相反,它们只是充当临床医务工作者在当前临床表现和社会心理背景下权衡个人从事自杀行为的相对风险的准则。

Factors that may increase risk or factors that may decrease risk are those that have been found to be statistically related to the presence or absence of suicidal behaviors. They do not necessarily impart a causal relationship. Rather they serve as guidelines for the clinician to weigh the relative risk of an individual engaging in suicide behaviors within the context of the current clinical presentation and psychosocial setting.

个体在危险和保护因素对其自杀行为倾向的影响程度上存在差异。每个危险和保护因素对其自杀的影响在他们的一生中都会有所不同。没有一个或一系列危险因素必然会导致自杀风险的增加。也没有一个或一系列保护性因素,可以确保防止自杀行为的发生。

Individuals differ in the degree to which risk and protective factors affect their propensity for engaging in suicidal behaviors. Within an individual, the contribution of each risk and protective factor to their suicidality will vary over the course of their lives. No one risk factor, or a set of risk factors, necessarily conveys increased suicide risk. Nor does one protective factor, or a set of protective factors, insures protection against engagement in suicidal behaviors.

此外,由于它们与自杀行为的统计相关性不同,因此这些因素并不相等,并且一个人无法"平衡"一组因素与另一组因素,以得出自杀风险的总和。一些危险因素是不可变的(如年龄、性别、种族/民族),而另一些危险因素则是针对特定情况而言(如房屋损失、慢性病引起的疼痛加剧以及精神病发作或加重)。

Furthermore, because of their different statistical correlations with suicide behaviors, these factors are not equal and one cannot "balance" one set of factors against another in order to derive a sum total score of relative suicide risk. Some risk factors are immutable (e.g., age, gender, race/ethnicity), while others are more situation-specific (e.g., loss of housing, exacerbation of pain in a chronic condition, and onset or exacerbation of psychiatric symptoms).

心理因素:

• 亲人、名人或同伴自杀;

• 自杀丧亲;

• 失去亲人(悲伤);

• 关系破裂(离婚,分居);

• 失去地位/尊严/职衔(公开的羞辱,被欺负或虐待,工作/任务失败)。

Psychological Factors:

• Suicide of a relative, someone famous, or a peer;

• Suicide bereavement;

• Loss of loved one (grief);

• Loss of relationship (divorce, separation);

• Loss of status/respect/rank (public humiliation, being bullied or abused, failure work/task).

社会因素：

• 有压力的生活事件(急性经历)；

• 失恋和其他重要关系的破裂；

• 其他事件(如被解雇，逮捕，驱逐，殴打)。

Social Factors：

• Stressful life events (acute experiences)；

• Breakups and other threats to prized relationships；

• Other events (e.g., fired, arrested, evicted, assaulted).

财务因素：

• 失业，不充分就业；

• 住房不稳定，无家可归；

• 债务过多，财务状况不佳(取消抵押品赎回权，赡养费，子女抚养费)。

Financial Factors：

• Unemployment, underemployment；

• Unstable housing, homeless；

• Excessive debt, poor finances (foreclosure, alimony, child support).

法律因素：

• 吸毒后驾驶/酒驾；

• 诉讼；

• 刑事犯罪和监禁。

Legal Factors：

• DUI/DWI；

• Lawsuit；

• Criminal offence and incarceration.

社会支持因素：

• 人际关系不佳(伴侣，父母，孩子)；

• 地理位置的疏离；

• 获得精神卫生保健的障碍；

• 最近的护理水平变化(出院)。

Social Support Factors：

• Poor interpersonal relationship (partner, parents, children)；

• Geographic isolation from support；

• Barriers to accessing mental health care；

• Recent change in level of care (discharge from inpatient psychiatry).

精神障碍因素：

• 情绪或情感障碍(重度抑郁,躁郁症,产后抑郁)；

• 人格障碍(尤其是边缘型和反社会型)；

• 精神分裂症；

• 焦虑症(创伤后应激障碍,恐慌)；

• 物质使用障碍(酒精,成瘾药物,尼古丁)；

• 饮食失调；

• 睡眠障碍或失调；

• 创伤(心理)。

Mental Disorders Factors：

• Mood or affective disorder (major depression, bipolar, post-partum)；

• Personality disorder (especially borderline and antisocial)；

• Schizophrenia；

• Anxiety (PTSD, panic)；

• Substance Use Disorder (alcohol, illicit drugs, nicotine)；

• Eating disorder；

• Sleep disturbance or disorder；

• Trauma (psychological).

医学因素：

• 脑外伤史(创伤性脑损伤)；

• 疾病晚期；

• 人类免疫缺陷病毒/获得性免疫缺陷综合征；

• 重大疾病的新诊断；

• 有健康问题；

• 慢性疾病恶化；

• 中毒；

• 物质戒断(酒精,鸦片,可卡因,安非他明)；

• 使用处方药提示自杀风险增加。

Medical Factors：

• History of Traumatic Brain Injury (TBI)；

• Terminal disease；

• HIV/AIDS；

• New diagnosis of major illness；

• Having a medical condition；

• Worsening of chronic illness；

- Intoxication;
- Substance withdrawal (alcohol, opiates, cocaine, amphetamines);
- Use of prescribed medication warning for increased risk of suicide.

身体症状因素：

- 慢性疼痛；
- 失眠；
- 功能限制。

Physical Symptoms Factors:

- Chronic pain;
- Insomnia;
- Function limitation.

已存在或不可改变的因素：

- 年龄；
- 性别；
- 种族；
- 婚姻状况（离婚，分居，丧偶）；
- 家族史；
- 自杀/自杀未遂；
- 精神疾病（包括冲动型人格障碍）；
- 虐待儿童——身体/心理/性；
- 性创伤；
- 较低的教育水平；
- 同性取向（女同/男同/双性恋者与跨性别族群）；
- 文化或宗教信仰。

Pre-existing & Non-modifiable Factors:

- Age;
- Gender;
- Race;
- Marital status (divorce, separate, widowed);
- Family history;
- Suicide/attempt;
- Mental illness (including SUD);
- Child maltreatment trauma—physical/psychological/sexual;
- Sexual trauma;
- Lower education level;

- Same sex orientation (LGBT);
- Cultural or religious beliefs.

2.2.2 自杀的保护因素

2.2.2 Protective Factors for Suicide

对保护因素的评估可以确定潜在的优势和适应力,用来减小自杀风险。了解保护因素可以成为处于危险中的人们获得希望的一种手段。应利用这些因素来减小短期和长期风险。

The assessment for protective factors can identify potential strengths and resiliency that may be used to buffer suicide risk. Recognizing protective factors can be a means to encourage hope among persons at risk. These factors should be capitalized upon to mitigate risk in both the short and long-term.

保护因素:

- 完整的社会支持;
- 积极的宗教信仰或信念(如果涉及行为的羞耻/内疚,也可能是一个危险因素);
- 婚姻和受抚养子女的存在;
- 与照顾者持续的支持关系;
- 积极的治疗性关系;
- 无抑郁症或物质滥用;
- 获得医疗和精神卫生资源;
- 冲动控制;
- 具有解决问题和应对问题的能力;
- 妊娠;
- 对生活满意;
- 自杀未遂后的情绪舒缓;
- "未竟事业"感;
- 良好的自尊、自信;
- 重要关系人对于患者自杀想法的认识;
- 归属感。

Protective Factors:

- Intact social supports;
- Active religious affiliation or faith (may also be a risk factor if shame/guilt about behaviour is involved);
- Marriage and presence of dependent children;

- Ongoing supportive relationship with a caregiver;
- Positive therapeutic relationship;
- Absence of depression or substance abuse;
- Access to medical and mental health resources;
- Impulse control;
- Proven problem-solving and coping skills;
- Pregnancy;
- Life satisfaction;
- Relief about not completing suicide;
- Sense of "unfinished business";
- Good self-esteem, self-confidence;
- Awareness of significant others about their suicidal thoughts;
- Sense of belonging.

帮助评估保护因素的问题例子：

- 你说你有自杀的想法，但没有付诸行动。到目前为止，是什么阻止了你？
- 生活中有什么让你想继续活下去？
- 在你的生活中，是谁让你想继续活下去？
- 当你感到不安全时，你会使用什么资源或你会向谁寻求帮助？
- 你曾经说过你没有对这些想法采取行动是因为什么。这个因素对你现在的决策有多大影响？
- 你对生活有什么期望或你想要实现什么目标？
- 当你感到挫败感时，你会使用什么解决问题或应对机制？
- 在过去，当你有自杀想法时，你和谁分享这些想法？
- 如果你是一个有精神信仰或宗教信仰的人，你的信仰是否起到了保护作用？如果是的话，是怎样起作用的？

Examples of Questions to Aid in the Assessment of Protective Factors:

- You say that you have had thoughts of suicide, but have not acted on them. What has stopped you thus far?
- What in life makes you want to keep on living?
- Who are the people in your life that make you want to go on living?
- What resources do you access when feeling unsafe or who are the people that you go to for support?
- You have said that in the past you didn't act on these thoughts because of X. How much is that factor into your decision-making now?
- What aspirations do you have for life or what goals would you like to accomplish?

• When feeling overwhelmed, what problem-solving mechanisms do you utilize?

• In the past when you had suicidal thoughts, with whom did you share these thoughts?

• If you are a spiritual or religious person, do your beliefs act as a protective factor and if so, how?

2.3 自杀风险的综合评估

2.3 Comprehensive Suicide Risk Assessment

确定自杀风险应包括三个任务:

①收集与患者从事自杀相关行为的意图有关的信息。

②评估可以提高或降低执行该意图的风险的因素。

③整合所有可用的信息,以确定风险水平,并给予适当的护理。

Determination of suicide risk should include three tasks:

①Gather information related to the patient's intent to engage in suicide-related behavior.

②Evaluate factors that elevate or reduce the risk of acting on that intent.

③Integrate all available information to determine the level of risk and appropriate setting for care.

理想情况下,应在任何自杀行为发生之前识别患者。尽早发现自杀意念为减少自杀未遂和死亡风险提供了最大的机会。我们了解自杀的连续性始于自杀的想法,演变为希望自己死亡,深化为行动意图,并制定了终结生命的方法或计划。

Ideally, a patient is identified before any suicidal behavior occurs. Early identification of suicide ideation presents the greatest opportunity to reduce the risk of suicide attempt and death. We understand the suicide continuum begins with suicide thoughts, evolving into a wish to die, consolidated into an intention to act, and resulting in a methodology or plan formulated to end one's life.

这些步骤的演变可能会持续数分钟或数年。连续过程中的每一步都提供了干预和预防自杀式暴力行为的机会。患者往往是在企图自杀后才被发现的。通常,评估个人自杀风险的第一次机会是由于护理人员、守门人或亲人识别出了警告信号。

The evolution of these steps can occur over minutes or years. Each step along the continuum presents an opportunity to intervene and prevent the act of suicide violence. All too often, a patient is identified after a suicide attempt is made. Often the first opportunity to assess an individual's suicide risk occurs because of the demonstration of warning signs that are identified by a caregiver, gatekeeper, or loved one.

识别警告信号是为早期评估和干预创造机会的关键。三种直接的警告信号特别能显示出自杀风险:口头或书面传达自杀想法;寻求获得枪支或药物等致命手段的途径;表现出准备行为,如将事情安排有序。如果出现一个或多个这种警告信号,就强烈表明需要进一步评估自杀风险。

Recognition of warning signs is the key to creating an opportunity for early assessment and intervention. Three direct warning signs are particularly indicative of suicide risk: communicating suicide thought verbally or in writing; seeking access to lethal means such as firearms or medications; and demonstrating preparatory behaviors such as putting affairs in order. Presence of one or more of these warning signs is a strong indication that further assessment is needed.

自杀风险评估不是绝对的。它没有明确的、有效的预测模型或风险分层定义。为简单起见,本书将推荐一个三级分层系统,来定义那些需要立即干预以预防自杀尝试行为。那些自杀行为风险较高的患者需要临床干预,那些自杀风险没有明显提高的人也可能从干预中受益。

Suicide risk assessment is not absolute. There are no clear, validated predictive models or risk stratification definitions. For simplicity's sake, this book will recommend a three-tier stratification system to define those patients in need of immediate intervention in order to prevent a suicide attempt. Those patients at an elevated risk of suicide behavior in the future are in need of a clinical intervention, and those for whom the risk of suicide is not significantly elevated may benefit from an intervention.

该指导手册阐述了急性风险的指定级别(高、中、低)分层。确定风险水平的重要性在于,它将为选择医疗机构、管理和后续治疗计划提供信息。

The stratification of assigned level of the acute risk (high, intermediate, and low) was elaborated by the instruction manual. The importance of determining the level of risk is that it will inform the decision regarding the choice of care setting, management and treatment plans to follow.

要记住的是,没有个体处于"没有自杀"风险的状态,因此,这种从没有绝对间断的连续性风险中强行划分的分层方法是不完美的。在住院期间进行的心理健康评估应包括全面的自杀风险评估,该评估在使用决策支持工具进行二次筛查之后实施。

It is worth remembering that no individual is at "no risk" of suicide, so these strata are an imperfect attempt to rationalize clear distinctions from within a continuum of risk with no absolute cutoffs. Mental health evaluations conducted during the hospitalization should include a comprehensive suicide risk assessment that goes beyond the secondary screening performed using the Decision Support Tool.

风险评估的目的是确定患者是否处于紧急危险中,并做出治疗决策。这也是与患者建立治疗关系的机会。全面的风险评估将有助于识别可能导致增加或减少自杀风险的危险性因素和保护性因素。

The purposes of the risk assessment are to determine whether the patient is in immediate danger and to make decisions about treatment. It is also an opportunity to form a therapeutic relationship with the patient. A complete risk assessment will help to identify both risk and protective factors that may contribute to an increased or decreased risk of suicide.

明确这些因素将帮助护士和医疗团队制定旨在加强或减轻可改变因素的干预措施,从而降低患者的自杀风险。各项风险评估的完成程度可能因环境和情况而异,但无论如何,必须确保患者安全,并应尽一切努力询问患者关于自杀意念和行为的情况。

Illuminating such factors will assist the nurse and health care team to develop interventions designed to strengthen or mitigate factors amendable to change, thus decreasing a patient's risk of suicide. The extent to which all components of the risk assessment are completed may vary depending on the setting and circumstances, but in any case the patient must be kept safe and all efforts should be made to inquire about suicide ideation and behaviour.

2.3.1 自杀风险评估流程

2.3.1 Process for Risk Assessment of Suicide

住院患者自杀风险评估包括三个步骤——初级筛查、二级筛查和自杀风险评估,三者是不同但相关的临床实践,旨在帮助卫生服务提供者了解患者自杀风险的性质。

Assessment of suicide risk for hospitalized patients includes three steps—primary screening, secondary screening, and suicide risk assessment. The three parts are distinct but related practices designed to help providers understand the nature of their patients's uicide risk.

初级筛查工具可用于检测所有住院患者(普遍筛查)或已知危险因素的患者(选择性筛查),如所有的抑郁症患者。初步筛查可通过口头进行(由筛查者提出问题)、使用铅笔和纸或者使用计算机实施。

Primary screening tools can be used to detect the presence of suicide risk in all patients (universal screening) or in patients with known risk factors (selective screening), such as all patients with depression. Primary screening may be conducted verbally (with the screener asking questions), using pencils and paper, or using a computer.

自杀风险评估是由训练有素的临床医生进行的全面评估,需要完成以下工作:

①确认可疑的自杀风险。

②根据患者的危险和保护因素以及其他信息来评估患者的直接危险。

③做出患者治疗计划的相关决策。

Suicide risk assessment is a comprehensive evaluation performed by a trained clinician to accomplish the following:

①Confirming suspected suicide risk.

②Estimating the immediate danger to the patient based on the patient's risk and protective factors and other information.

③Deciding on a course of treatment.

风险评估包括结构化问卷和与患者及其支持者进行开放式的对话,以了解患者的思想、行为、危险因素(如获取致命手段的途径或自杀未遂史)、保护性因素(如直系亲属的支持),以及医疗和精神健康史。

Risk assessments can involve structured questionnaires or be open-ended conversations with patients and their supports to gain insight into the patient's thoughts and behavior, risk factors (e.g., access to lethal means or a history of suicide attempts), protective factors (e.g., immediate family support), and medical and mental health history.

一个人的自杀风险是动态的:随着时间的推移,根据情感状态、生活事件以及危险和保护因素的复杂相互作用而变化。这些因素的评估在总体评估中起着重要作用。

A person's risk for suicide is dynamic: changing over time based on affective states, life events, and the complex interplay of risk and protective factors. Evaluation of these factors plays an important role in the overall assessment.

自杀风险评估必须包括对患者内部经历、思想、信念和态度的评估,他们的外部关系和压力源,以及增加自杀可能性和阻止其采取行动的各种因素。临床医生必须整合所有这些数据,最终通过临床判断来制定风险评估和治疗计划。

A suicide risk assessment must include the evaluation of the patient's internal experience, thoughts, beliefs, and attitudes; their external world of relationships and stressors; as well as the myriad of factors that increase the likelihood of suicide and those that prevent them from action. All of these data must then be integrated by the clinician who must ultimately use clinical judgment to formulate a risk assessment and treatment plan.

对患者自杀风险的评估通常是在危机发生期间进行的,在此期间,该人可能会感到威胁,认为他/她分享自杀想法和行为将导致住院期间自主权丧失、行为受限或被认为有精神疾病及有关污名导致自尊丧失。如果这类患者试图将其症状减轻到最轻程度以便出院,或者使亲人或临床医生放心,则这种危机可能会扰乱风险评估。

The evaluation of a patient's risk for suicide is often performed during a time of crisis during which the person may feel threatened that his/her sharing of suicidal thoughts and behaviors will result in the loss of autonomy through hospitalization, behavioral restriction, or the loss of esteem through recognition of psychiatric illness and the associated stigma. This crisis may confound the risk assessment if the identified patient seeks to minimize her/his symptoms in order to be released, or to reassure loved ones or the clinician.

耻辱感可能会阻止那些有自杀倾向和有自我指向暴力行为的人寻求帮助。因此,对于临床医务工作者而言,重要的是要意识到潜在的患者,尽量减少他们的自杀风险,并试图安抚和说服临床医务工作者他们可以出院治疗。

Stigma may play a role in discouraging help-seeking behavior for those at risk for suicide and self-directed violence. It is therefore important for clinicians to be aware of the potential for patients to minimize their suicide risks and try to reassure and convince the clinician they can be released from care.

有自杀危机的患者通常会感到非常羞耻,并且往往对判断非常敏感。因此,中立的、非判断性的评估更有可能得出可靠的数据并促进与患者的合作。评估应该是循序渐进的,从一般问题到具体问题。如果自杀危险因素变得明显,则需要进行更详细的研究。

Patients in a suicide crisis often feel a great degree of shame and tend to be exquisitely sensitive to being judged. Therefore, a neutral, non-judgmental assessment is more likely to elicit reliable data and foster an alliance with the patient. The assessment should be stepwise, from general to specific questions. More detailed exploration is indicated if risk factors for suicide become apparent.

重要的是要认识到那些没有明确表达想法或计划、寻找手段的人,自杀风险仍然很高。真正打算终止生命的人可能会掩盖警告信号。如果患者不愿或无法提供准确的信息，临床医务工作者可能需要依赖客观观察和论证行为。在这种情况下，建议咨询心理健康专业人员。

It is important to recognize that risk may still be high in persons who are not explicitly expressing ideation or plans, searching for means. Persons who may truly intend to end their lives may conceal warning signs. If the patient is not willing or able to provide accurate information, then the clinician may need to relay on objective observations and demonstrated behaviors. Consultation with mental health professionals is advisable in such instances.

一些医疗卫生服务提供者担心，询问有关自杀的问题可能会促使患者产生自杀意念。但是，有证据表明对自杀意念和意图的直接评估并不会增加自杀风险。谈论它不会导致自杀倾向；如果回避这个话题，则有可能忽略或遗漏自杀倾向。应该以非判断性的方式来构想问题，以提高获取真实回答的可能性。

Some providers fear that by asking about suicide they may prompt the patient to feel suicidal. However, evidence shows that direct assessment of suicide ideation and intent does not increase the risk for suicide. There is no risk of causing suicidality by talking about it; there is a risk of ignoring or missing suicidality if the topic is avoided. Questions should be framed in a non-judgmental way to enhance the probability of eliciting a truthful response.

2.3.2 风险评估要素

2.3.2 Elements of Risk Assessment

（1）进行精神病学评估。
- 存在的问题——从患者的角度出发，包括确定的社会心理压力源；
- 现病史——症状的持续时间和严重程度；
- 既往精神病史——过去的精神病住院、日期、地点、诊断；
- 既往病史——疾病、手术、日期和住院地点；
- 目前和过去的药物；
- 药物过敏；
- 物质使用史——当前和过去的使用情况、日期和治疗机构的地点、戒断史；
- 法证史——指控、假释、缓刑、监禁时间；
- 家族史——精神疾病、自杀未遂、自杀死亡；
- 社会心理史——情感和性虐待、教育、职业、人际关系、非正式和正式支持网络；
- 护理诊断。

（1）Conduct a Psychiatric Assessment.

• Presenting problem—from the perspective of the patient, including identified psychosocial stressors;

• History of present illness—duration and severity of symptoms;

• Past psychiatric history—past psychiatric hospitalizations, dates, locations, diagnoses;

• Past medical history—illnesses, surgeries, dates and locations of hospitalizations;

• Current and past medications;

• Drug allergies;

• Substance use history—current and past use of all substances, dates and locations of treatment settings, history of withdrawal;

• Forensic history—past and current charges, parole, probation, jail time;

• Family history—mental illness, suicide attempts, death by suicide;

• Psychosocial history—emotional and sexual abuse, education, occupation, relationships, informal and formal support networks;

• Nursing diagnosis.

（2）关于自杀意念和自杀行为的调查。

• 自杀意念——询问患者关于生死观的不正常想法。患者是否正在考虑自杀？

• 自杀计划——询问自杀计划。患者是否选择或考虑了自杀的方法？如果是的话,患者采取措施来实施计划了吗？

• 获得手段——患者是否能够获得所选择的方法？选择的计划是否合理？对于患者来说,获得这些手段或实施计划有多容易？

• 意图——患者是否打算死亡？患者对死亡的渴望有多强烈？患者是否已经为死亡做好准备,例如处理后事或写遗书？这个人有没有采取措施尽量减少被发现？这个人在试图自杀之前是否寻求过帮助？

• 致命性——询问方法以确定致命性。患者是否相信所选择的方法是致命的？所选择的方法和计划是否考虑到干扰？

• 保护因素——是否有什么人或环境使得患者想要继续活下去？有什么障碍阻止患者自杀吗？

• 以前的尝试行为——病人是否曾有过自杀未遂？如果是的话,促发因素是什么？每次尝试行为是什么时候发生的？方法是什么？医疗严重程度是多少？是否与酒精或毒品有关？

（2）Inquire about Suicide Ideation and Behaviour.

• Suicide ideation—Ask the patient questions to illicit information about their thoughts on living and dying. Is the patient thinking about killing oneself?

　•　Plan—Inquire about a suicide plan. Has the patient chosen a method or considered options to kill oneself? If so, has the person taken steps to put the plan in place?

　•　Access to Means—Does the patient have access to the chosen method? Is the chosen plan plausible? How easy would it be for the patient to access such means or put plans in place?

　•　Intent—Does the patient intend to die? What is the intensity of the patients desire to die? Has the patient made preparations for death, such as putting affairs in order, or writing a suicide note? Has the person taken steps to minimize being discovered? Has the person sought help prior to attempting suicide?

　•　Lethality—Inquire about methods to determine lethality. Did the patient believe that the chosen method would be lethal? Would the chosen method and plan allow for intervention?

　•　Protective factors—Are there any people or circumstances that allow the patient to want to go on living? Are there any barriers that prevent the patient from taking their life?

　•　Previous attempts—Has the patient had past suicide attempts? If so, what were the precipitants? When did each attempt occur? What was the method? What was the medical severity? Were alcohol or drugs involved?

2.3.3 间接信息来源

2.3.3 Indirect Sources of Information

间接信息是对所有成年患者进行自杀风险评估的一个重要组成部分,尤其是在护士不认识患者,不愿或无法参与自杀风险评估的情况下。间接信息是指从了解患者的其他人那里获得的信息,如家庭、其他重要的人。

Collateral information is an important component of a suicide risk assessment with all adult clients, particularly in cases where the client is unknown to the nurse, unwilling or unable to participate in suicide risk assessment. Collateral information is what is obtained from others who know the client, such as family and significant others.

这些信息可以提供关于患者的精神状态或行为的重要信息,这些信息可能暗示着自杀意念,以及最近可能对患者产生影响的任何压力源。

Such information can provide important information about the client's mental state or behaviour that may indicate suicide ideation, as well as any recent stressors that may be impacting on the client.

获取间接信息的问题例子：

①他们和平时表现一样吗？

②他们有没有说过他们"死了会更好"？

③有没有关于"事情很快就会变好"的说法？

④你担心过他们吗？ 他们看起来是沮丧还是抑郁？

⑤他们比平时饮酒更多吗？

Examples of questions for acquiring collateral:

①Are they their usual self?

②Have they made any comments that they would be "better off dead"?

③Have there been any statements about "things getting better soon"?

④Have you been worried about them? Do they seem down or depressed?

⑤Are they drinking more than usual?

2.3.4 自杀风险评估的不同方面

2.3.4 Different Aspects of Suicide Risk Assessment

（1）全面的精神评估。

（1）Comprehensive Mental Assessment.

考虑自杀与精神疾病之间的重要关系，自杀评估的一个主要部分是一项全面的精神/社会心理评估，以收集有关信息。

Given the significant association between suicide and mental illness, a major part of suicide assessment is a comprehensive psychiatric/psychosocial assessment to gather information regarding.

在精神/社会心理评估中，心理状态测试是评估个体当前心理状态的一种系统方法，特别是有关心理、情绪、社会和神经功能。

Within the psychiatric/psychosocial assessment, a mental status exam is a systematic approach to the assessment of an individual's current mental status, specifically related to psychological, emotional, social, and neurologic functioning.

确定与自杀或其他自杀行为风险增加相关的特定精神体征和症状也是很重要的。与自杀未遂或自杀相关的症状包括攻击、对他人的暴力、冲动、绝望和激动。

It is also important to identify specific psychiatric signs and symptoms that are correlated with an increased risk of suicide or other suicidal behaviors. Symptoms that have been associated with suicide attempts or with suicide include aggression, violence toward others, impulsiveness, hopelessness and agitation.

精神焦虑被定义为焦虑、恐惧或忧虑的主观感觉，无论是否有具体的对象，它也与自杀风险增加有关，例如快感缺失、彻底失眠和惊恐发作。

Psychic anxiety, which has been defined as subjective feelings of anxiety, fearfulness, or apprehension whether or not focused on specific concerns, has also been associated with an increased risk of suicide, as have anhedonia, global insomnia, and panic attacks.

在精神疾病评估中，确认家族史尤为重要。精神科医生应特别询问是否有自杀和自杀未遂以及任何精神疾病住院史或精神疾病（包括物质使用障碍）的家族史。当自杀发生在直系家属身上时，了解更多的情况通常是有帮助的，包括患者的参与以及患者和亲属在自杀时的年龄。

Identifying family history is particularly important during the psychiatric evaluation. The psychiatrist should specifically inquire about the presence of suicide and suicide attempts as well as a family history of any psychiatric hospitalizations or mental illness, including substance use disorders. When suicides have occurred in firstdegree relatives, it is often helpful to learn more about the circumstances, including the patient's involvement and the patient's and relative's ages at the time of the suicide.

患者的童年和目前的家庭环境也是相关的，因为家庭功能障碍的许多方面可能与自我毁灭行为有关。这些因素包括家庭冲突或分居史、父母法律纠纷、家庭药物使用、家庭暴力以及身体或性虐待。

The patient's childhood and current family milieu are also relevant, since many aspects of family dysfunction may be linked to self-destructive behaviors. Such factors include a history of family conflict or separation, parental legal trouble, family substance use, domestic violence, and physical or sexual abuse.

对患者目前的心理社会状况进行评估对于发现可能增加自杀风险的急性社会心理危机或慢性心理压力源非常重要（如经济或法律困难、人际冲突或损失、男女同性恋或双性恋青年的压力源、住房问题、失业、教育失败）。其他重要的诱因包括感知损失、最近或即将遭受的羞辱。

An assessment of the patient's current psychosocial situation is important to detect acute psychosocial crises or chronic psychosocial stressors that may augment suicide risk (e.g., financial or legal difficulties; interpersonal conflicts or losses; stressors in gay, lesbian, or bisexual youths; housing problems; job loss; educational failure). Other significant precipitants may include perceived losses or recent or impending humiliation.

临床医生需要了解患者的优势和弱点。特殊的优势和弱点包括应对技能、人格特征、思维方式以及发展和心理需求等因素。例如,除了作为依赖状态的症状外,绝望、攻击和冲动也可能构成特征,这些特征很大程度上与增加自杀行为的风险有关。

The clinician needs to appreciate the strengths and vulnerabilities of the individual patient. Particular strengths and vulnerabilities may include such factors as coping skills, personality traits, thinking styles, and developmental and psychological needs. For example, in addition to serving as state-dependent symptoms, hopelessness, aggression, and impulsivity may also constitute traits, greater degrees of which may be associated with an increased risk for suicide behaviors.

增加的自杀风险也出现在那些思维极端或思维两极分化的人以及思想封闭的人身上(如视角狭窄和兴趣集中)。自我期望值过高的完美主义是临床实践中发现的另一个可能导致自杀风险的因素。

Increased suicide risk has also been seen in individuals who exhibit thought constriction or polarized thinking as well in individuals with closed-mindedness (i.e., a narrowed scope and intensity of interests). Perfectionism with excessively high self-expectation is another factor that has been noted in clinical practice to be a possible contributor to suicide risk.

在权衡个别患者的优势和弱点时,也有助于确定患者从事冒险行为的倾向以及患者过去对压力的反应,包括现实检验能力和忍受拒绝的能力、主观的孤独,或当他/她的独特心理需求没有得到满足时的心理痛苦。

In weighing the strengths and vulnerabilities of the individual patient, it is also helpful to determine the patient's tendency to engage in risk-taking behaviors as well as the patient's past responses to stress, including the capacity for reality testing and the ability to tolerate rejection, subjective loneliness, or psychological pain when his or her unique psychological needs are not met.

了解患者的心理社会状况对评估自杀风险和制定治疗方案也是至关重要的,并帮助患者调动外部支持,这可以对自杀风险起到保护作用。

An understanding of the patient's psychosocial situation is also essential in estimating suicide risk and formulating a treatment plan, and helping the patient to mobilize external supports, which can have a protective influence on suicide risk.

(2)询问自杀的想法、计划、行为。

(2)Ask about Suicide Thoughts, Plans, Behaviors.

评估自杀意图和自杀意图的程度是评估过程的关键组成部分。自杀风险临床评估的第一个方面是对患者的自杀想法、根据这些想法采取行动的意愿以及患者不从事自杀行为的意愿或能力的评估。

Assessing for current intent and the degree of intent for suicide is a key component of the assessment process. The first aspect of the clinical assessment of suicide risk is the evaluation of the patient's thoughts of suicide, the intention to act on those thoughts, and the desire or the ability of the patient to not engage in suicide behaviors.

任何有自杀倾向的行为证据都暗含更高的风险水平。自杀准备行为包括制定终止生命的计划、排练计划或采取步骤为自杀尝试行为做准备(如存放药物,购买枪支,将绳索绑在套索上)。评估计划的致命性很重要,但患者对致命性的估计以及对其行动或潜在行动可能后果的理解同样重要。

Any evidence of action toward a suicide attempt suggests a higher level of risk. Suicide preparatory behaviors include the development of a plan to end one's life, rehearsing a plan, or taking steps to prepare for an attempt (e.g., stockpiling medications, buying a gun, tying a rope into a noose). Assessing the lethality of the plan is important, but also important is the patient's estimation of the lethality and understanding of the probable consequences of his/her actions or potential actions.

许多自杀的人可能会透露想要从事自杀行为的警示迹象或信号。这些警告信号是对与自杀行为最密切相关的情绪、想法或行为的观察,反映了即将发生的风险。

Many suicidal individuals may reveal warning signs or signals of their intention to engage suicide behaviors. These warning signs are observations of precipitating emotions, thoughts, or behaviors that are most proximally associated with a suicide act and reflect imminent risk.

过去的自杀未遂史是自杀最重要的危险因素之一,更严重、更频繁或更近期的尝试行为可能会增加这种风险。因此,对临床医务工作者来说,询问过去的自杀未遂和自我毁灭行为是非常重要的,包括对自杀未遂的具体询问。

A history of past suicide attempts is one of the most significant risk factors for suicide, and this risk may be increased by more serious, more frequent, or more recent attempts. Therefore, it is important for the clinicians to inquire about past suicide attempts and self-destructive behaviors, including specific questioning about aborted suicide attempts.

对于每一次的尝试行为或中止的尝试行为,临床医务工作者应设法获取关于诱因、时间、意图、后果以及自杀未遂的医疗严重程度的细节。应确定患者在试图自杀之前酒精和药物的摄入量,因为醉酒可能会增加自杀企图的冲动性,但这也可能是更严重的自杀计划的一个组成部分。

For each attempt or aborted attempt, the clinicians should try to obtain details about the precipitants, timing, intent, and consequences as well as the attempt's medical severity. The patient's consumption of alcohol and drugs before the attempt should also be ascertained, since intoxication can facilitate impulsive suicide attempts but can also be a component of a more serious suicide plan.

在了解最终导致自杀未遂的问题时,还应描述关于自杀未遂人际关系方面的内容。例如,导致尝试行为的动力或人际关系问题、自杀时出现的人员、与其交流过自杀的人员以及那次尝试行为是如何避免的。

In understanding the issues that culminated in the suicide attempt, interpersonal aspects of the attempt should also be delineated. Examples might include the dynamic or interpersonal issues leading up to the attempt, significant persons present at the time of the attempt, persons to whom the attempt was communicated, and how the attempt was averted.

确定患者对自杀企图的想法也很重要,例如他/她自己对所选择方法致命性的理解、对生活的矛盾心理、对自杀场景的预想、预谋程度、自杀意念的持续存在以及对自杀企图的反应。询问过去的冒险行为也很有帮助,如不安全的性行为和鲁莽驾驶。

It is also important to determine the patient's thoughts about the attempt, such as his or her own perception of the chosen method's lethality, ambivalence toward living, visualization of death, degree of premeditation, persistence of suicide ideation, and reaction to the attempt. It is also helpful to inquire about past risk-taking behaviors such as unsafe sexual practices and reckless driving.

一般来说,一个人对自杀的想法越多,制定了具体的自杀计划,并打算按照这些计划采取行动,那么他/她的自杀风险就越大。因此,作为自杀评估的一部分,有必要特别询问患者的自杀想法、计划、行为和意图。

In general, the more an individual has thought about suicide, has made specific plans for suicide, and intends to act on those plans, the greater will be his or her risk. Thus, as part of the suicide assessment it is essential to inquire specifically about the patient's suicidal thoughts, plans, behaviors, and intent.

虽然这些问题通常会自然地从患者现状的讨论中产生,但这并不一定是真的。问题的确切措辞和提问的范围也会因临床情况而异。

Although such questions will often flow naturally from discussion of the patient's current situation, this will not invariably be true. The exact wording of questions and the extent of questioning will also differ with the clinical situation.

询问自杀意念是自杀评估的重要组成部分。虽然有些人担心提出自杀的话题会把这个问题"植入"患者的脑海,但事实并非如此。事实上,对自杀患者来说,提出自杀意念的话题可能是一种宽慰,为他/她打开了一条讨论的途径,给予了他/她一个被理解的机会。

Inquiring about suicide ideation is an essential component of the suicide assessment. Although some fear that raising the topic of suicide will "plant" the issue in the patient's mind, this is not the case. In fact, broaching the issue of suicide ideation may be a relief for the suicide patient by opening an avenue for discussion and giving him or her an opportunity to feel understood.

在询问关于自杀的想法时,从患者对生活的感受开始提问通常是有帮助的,比如"在这个时候,生活对你来说是怎样的?"或者"你是否曾觉得生活不值得过下去?"或者"你是否曾希望自己能沉睡而不醒来?"

In asking about suicide ideas, it is often helpful to begin with questions that address the patient's feelings about living, such as, "How does life seem to you at this point?" or "Have you ever felt that life was not worth living?" or "Did you ever wish you could go to sleep and just not wake up?"

如果患者的反应反映出对生活不满或想要逃避生活,这种反应自然会导致更具体的问题,如患者是否有过死亡或自杀的想法。当这些想法被激发时,重点关注它们的性质、频率、范围和时间,并了解它们发生时的人际关系、情境和症状。

If the patient's response reflects dissatisfaction with life or a desire to escape it, this response can lead naturally into more specific questions about whether the patient has had thoughts of death or suicide. When such thoughts are elicited, it is important to focus on the nature, frequency, extent, and timing of them and to understand the interpersonal, situational, and symptomatic context in which they are occurring.

即使患者最初否认死亡或自杀的想法,精神疾病学家也应该考虑询问更多的问题。例如询问对未来的计划或者近期自我伤害的行为或想法。

Even if the patient initially denies thoughts of death or suicide, the psychiatrist should consider asking additional questions. Examples might include asking about plans for the future or about recent acts or thoughts of self-harm.

不管访谈的方式如何,即使有这样的想法,并不是所有人都会报告自己有自杀的想法。因此,根据临床情况,精神疾病医生与患者的家人或朋友交谈以确定他们是否观察到这些行为或知道患者有暗示自杀倾向的想法是很重要的。

Regardless of the approach to the interview, not all individuals will report having suicide ideas even when such thoughts are present. Thus, depending on the clinical circumstances, it may be important for the psychiatrist to speak with family members or friends to determine whether they have observed behavior or have been privy to thoughts that suggest suicide ideation.

如果存在自杀想法,精神疾病学家需进一步调查更多关于自杀具体计划的详细信息,以及为实施这些计划而采取的任何步骤。虽然一些自杀行为可能在很少或没有计划的情况下冲动发生,但更详细的计划通常与更大的自杀风险有关。需要特别注意暴力和不可逆转的方法,如火器、跳楼和机动车事故。然而,患者对该方法致命性的看法可能与该方法本身的实际致命性同样重要。

If suicide ideation is present, the psychiatrist will next probe for more detailed information about specific plans for suicide and any steps that have been taken toward enacting those plans. Although some suicide acts can occur impulsively with little or no planning, more detailed plans are generally associated with a greater suicide risk. Violent and irreversible methods, such as firearms, jumping, and motor vehicle accidents, require particular attention. However, the patient's belief about the lethality of the method may be as important as the actual lethality of the method itself.

无论患者是否制定了自杀计划都应探讨患者的自杀意图。自杀意图反映了患者死亡意愿的强烈程度,可以通过确定患者的自杀动机以及自杀目标的严重程度来评估,包括任何与自杀有关的行为或计划。该计划的致命性可以通过有关方法的问题、患者使用该计划的知识和技能以及干预人员或保护性环境的缺乏来确定。

Regardless of whether the patient has developed a suicide plan, the patient's level of suicide intent should be explored. Suicide intent reflects the intensity of a patient's wish to die and can be assessed by determining the patient's motivation for suicide as well as the seriousness and extent of his or her aim to die, including any associated behaviors or planning for suicide. The lethality of the plan can be ascertained through questions about the method, the patient's knowledge and skill concerning its use, and the absence of intervening persons or protective circumstances.

一般来说,意图越强烈越清晰,自杀的风险就越高,因此,即使是一个具有低致命性自杀计划或自杀未遂的患者,如果自杀意图强烈且患者相信所选择的方法将是致命的,那么将来他也可能处于高风险之中。同时,低自杀意图的患者仍然可能因错误地认为某一特定方法不是致命的而死于自杀。

In general, the greater and clearer the intent, the higher the risk for suicide will be. Thus, even a patient with a low lethality suicide plan or attempt may be at a high risk in the future if intentions are strong and the patient believes that the chosen method will be fatal. At the same time, a patient with low suicide intent may still die from suicide by erroneously believing that a particular method is not lethal.

如果患者没有报告计划,精神科医生可以询问患者在什么情况下会考虑自杀(如离婚、入狱、住房损失)或在不久的将来是否会制定或实施这样的计划。如果患者报告说他或她不太可能对自杀的想法采取行动,精神疾病学家应该确定是什么因素导致了这种预期,从而可以确定保护因素。

If the patient does not report a plan, the psychiatrist can ask whether there are certain conditions under which the patient would consider suicide (e.g., divorce, going to jail, housing loss) or whether it is likely that such a plan will be formed or acted on in the near future. If the patient reports that he or she is unlikely to act on the suicide thoughts, the psychiatrist should determine what factors are contributing to that expectation, as such questioning can identify protective factors.

可能有助于询问自杀想法、计划和行为的具体方面的问题:

Questions that may be helpful in inquiring about specific aspects of suicide thoughts, plans and behaviors:

• 你是否曾觉得生活不值得过下去?

• 你是否曾希望自己能入睡而永远不醒来呢?

• Have you ever felt that life was not worth living?

• Did you ever wish you could go to sleep and just not wake up?

跟进询问有关死亡、自残或自杀的具体问题:

Follow up with specific questions that ask about thoughts of death, self-harm, or suicide:

• 你最近想过死亡吗?

• 有没有事情让你想要伤害自己?

• 你是什么时候开始有这种想法的?

• 导致这种想法的原因有哪些(如人际和社会心理因素,包括真实或想象中的损失;具体的症状如情绪变化、快感缺失、绝望、焦虑、激惹、精神疾病)?

• 这些想法多久发生一次(包括频率、强迫性、可控性)?

• 你已经开始按那些想法行事了吗?

• 你认为你将来有多大可能会采取行动?

• 你是否曾经开始伤害(或杀死)自己,由于某种原因停止了(例如,拿着刀对着你的身体,但在行动之前停下来,或是去桥边但没有跳进河里)?

• 如果你真的自杀了,你想象会发生什么(例如,逃跑、与其他重要的人团聚、重生、其他人的反应)?

• 你是否制定了一个自伤或自杀的具体计划?(如果有,计划包括什么?)

• 你有准备工具吗?

• 你是否做过任何特别的准备(例如,购买特定物品、写便条或遗嘱、做财务安排、采取措施以避免被发现、排练计划)?

• 你和别人谈过你的计划吗?

• 你的未来是什么样子的?

• 什么事情会让你对未来有更多的(或更少的)希望(例如,治疗、关系协调、压力源解决)?

• 什么事情会让你尝试自杀的可能性更大(或更小)?

• 你的生活中有什么事情会导致你想逃避生活或死亡?

• 生活中有哪些事情让你想要继续活下去?

• 如果你开始有再次伤害自己或自杀的想法,你会怎么做?

• Is death something you've thought about recently?

• Have things ever reached the point that you've thought of harming yourself?

• When did you first notice such thoughts?

• What led up to the thoughts (e.g., interpersonal and psychosocial precipitants, including real or imagined losses; specific symptoms such as mood changes, anhedonia, hopelessness, anxiety, agitation, psychosis)?

• How often have those thoughts occurred (including frequency, obsessional quality, controllability)?

• How close have you come to acting on those thoughts?

• How likely do you think it is that you will act on them in the future?

• Have you ever started to harm (or kill) yourself but stopped before doing something (e.g., holding a knife to your body but stopping before acting, going to the edge of a bridge but not jumping)?

• What do you envision happening if you actually killed yourself (e.g., escaping, reunioning with significant others, rebirth, reactions of others)?

• Have you made a specific plan to harm or kill yourself? (If so, what does the plan include?)

• Do you have weapons available to you?

• Have you made any particular preparations (e.g., purchasing specific items, writing a note or a will, making financial arrangements, taking steps to avoid discovery, rehearsing the plan)?

• Have you spoken to anyone about your plans?

• How does the future look to you?

• What things would lead you to feel more (or less) hopeful about the future (e.g., treatment, reconciliation of relationship, resolution of stressors)?

• What things would make it more (or less) likely that you would try to kill yourself?

• What things in your life would lead you to want to escape from life or be dead?

• What things in your life make you want to go on living?

• If you began to have thoughts of harming or killing yourself again, what would you do?

对自杀未遂或有自伤行为的个人通常还可以询问以下问题:

For individuals who have attempted suicide or engaged in self-damaging actions, additional questions can be asked in general terms:

• 你能否描述发生了什么吗(例如,环境、起因、对未来的看法、酒精或其他物质的使用、伤害的严重性)?

• 你在尝试之前有什么想法?

• 你认为会发生什么(例如,沉睡还是受伤还是死亡,或从某个特定的人那里得到反应)?

• 当时还有其他人在场吗?

• 事后你是自己寻求帮助,还是有人为你寻求帮助?

• 你是打算被人发现,还是偶然被发现的?

• 事后你有什么感觉(例如,解脱还是后悔活着)?

• 事后你是否接受过治疗(例如,药物疗法还是精神治疗,急诊、住院还是门诊)?

• 尝试自杀之后,你对事物的看法有没有改变,或者有什么不同?

• 过去你有没有尝试过伤害(或杀死)自己?

• Can you describe what happened (e.g., circumstances, precipitants, view of future, use of alcohol or other substances, seriousness of injury)?

• What thoughts were you having beforehand that led up to the attempt?

• What did you think would happen (e.g., going to sleep versus injury versus dying, getting a reaction out of a particular person)?

• Were other people present at the time?

• Did you seek help afterward yourself, or did someone get help for you?

• Had you planned to be discovered, or were you found accidentally?

• How did you feel afterward (e.g., relief versus regret at being alive)?

• Did you receive treatment afterward (e.g., medical versus psychiatric, emergency department versus inpatient versus outpatient)?

• Has your view of things changed, or is there anything different for you since the attempt?

• Are there other times in the past when you've tried to harm (or kill) yourself?

对于有反复自杀想法或未遂的人,可以询问以下问题:

For individuals with repeated suicide thoughts or attempts, additional questions can be asked:

• 你有多少次试图伤害自己(或自杀)?

• 最近一次是什么时候?

• 你能描述一下你最想自杀时的想法吗?

• 你最严重的自杀或自杀未遂发生在什么时候?

• 是什么导致了这一切,后来又发生了什么?

• About how often have you tried to harm (or kill) yourself?

• When was the most recent time?

• Can you describe your thoughts at the time that you were thinking most seriously about suicide?

• When was your most serious attempt at harming or killing yourself?

• What led up to it, and what happened afterward?

对于有精神疾病的人,要特别询问幻觉和妄想:

For individuals with psychosis, ask specifically about hallucinations and delusions:

• 你能描述一下这些声音吗(例如,单一的还是多重的、男性的还是女性的、内部的还是外部的、可识别的还是不可识别的)?

• 这些声音都说了什么(例如,积极的评论、消极的评论还是威胁? 如果这些评论是命令,确定它们是无害的还是有害的,请举例)?

• 你如何应对(或回应)这些声音?

• 你做过哪些声音让你做的事吗?(是什么使你听从这些声音的? 如果你试图抵制它们,是什么让抵制变得困难?)

• 曾经有过声音告诉你伤害自己或自杀吗?(多久一次? 发生了什么?)

• 你是担心得了重病还是你的身体在退化?

• 即使别人告诉你没有什么可担心的,你也担心自己的财务状况吗?

• 有什么事情让你感到愧疚或自责吗?

• Can you describe the voices (e.g., single versus multiple, male versus female, internal versus external, recognizable versus nonrecognizable)?

• What do the voices say (e.g., positive remarks versus negative remarks versus threats? If the remarks are commands, determine if they are for harmless versus harmful acts; ask for examples)?

• How do you cope with (or respond to) the voices?

• Have you ever done what the voices ask you to do? (What led you to obey the voices? If you tried to resist them, what made it difficult?)

• Have there been times when the voices told you to hurt or kill yourself? (How often? What happened?)

• Are you worried about having a serious illness or that your body is rotting?

• Are you concerned about your financial situation even when others tell you there's nothing to worry about?

• Are there things that you've been feeling guilty about or blaming yourself for?

考虑评估患者除了伤害自己之外,还有可能伤害他人的可能性:

Consider assessing the patient's potential to harm others in addition to him－or herself:

• 你认为还有其他人可能对你所经历的事情负责吗(例如,迫害的想法、被动的经历)?

• 你有伤害他们的想法吗?

• 你还想和其他人一起死吗?

• 有没有你认为没有你就无法继续生活下去的人?

• Are there others who you think may be responsible for what you're experiencing (e.g., persecutory ideas, passivity experiences)?

• Are you having any thoughts of harming them?

• Are there other people you would want to die with you?

• Are there others who you think would be unable to go on without you?

三个直接警告信号预示着在不久的将来自杀行为发生的可能性最高。观察到这些警告信号需要立即引起注意,进行心理健康评估、转诊或考虑住院,以确保个人的安全、稳定和保障。

Three direct warning signs portend the highest likelihood of suicidal behaviors occurring in the near future. Observing these warning signs warrants immediate attention, mental health evaluation, referral, or consideration of hospitalization to ensure the safety, stability and security of the individual.

自杀式交流——撰写或谈论自杀,希望死亡(威胁要伤害或杀死自己)或有意采取上述行动的意图;

Suicide Communication—writing or talking about suicide, wish to die (threatening to hurt or kill self) or intention to act on those ideas;

自杀准备——自杀意图的证据或表达,或采取措施实施计划;为需要抚养的

人(孩子、宠物、老人)作出安排,或进行其他准备工作,例如更新遗嘱,安排财产,与所爱的人道别等;

Preparations for Suicide—evidence or expression of suicide intent, or taking steps towards implementation of a plan; making arrangements to divest responsibility for dependent others (children, pets, elders), or making other preparations such as updating wills, making financial arrangements for paying bills, saying goodbye to loved ones, etc;

寻求获取或近期使用致命手段——例如武器、药物、毒素或其他致命手段。

Seeking Access or Recent Use of Lethal Means—such as weapons, medications, toxins or other lethal means.

如果此人以前有过自杀未遂的经历,有自杀家族史或打算使用具有致命性的方法,则这些信号可能会预示自杀风险更大。

These signals are likely to be even more dangerous if the person has previously attempted suicide, has a family history of suicide or intends to use a method that is lethal.

一旦评估了患者的自杀意念、意图和行为,就应系统地考虑影响风险的其他因素,以最终确定风险水平。这些因素可能包括危险以及保护因素,如果可以改变,可能会成为减少自杀风险的临床干预重点。

Once the patient's suicidal ideation, intent and behaviors are assessed then other factors that influence risk should be considered in a systematic way to finalize the determination of risk level. These factors may include risk as well as protective factors that, if modifiable, could become the focus of clinical intervention to reduce the risk for suicide.

危险因素——增加自杀行为的可能性,包括可改变和不可改变的指标;

Risk Factors—increasing the likelihood of suicide behavior and including modifiable and non-modifiable indicators;

保护因素——能力、素质、环境和个人资源,增强适应力,促使个体走向成长、稳定和健康,增强应对不同生活事件的能力和减少自杀行为的可能性。

Protective Factors—capacities, qualities, environmental and personal resources that increase resilience, driving individuals towards growth, stability and health, and increasing the ability to cope with different life events and decreasing the likelihood of suicidal behavior.

仅凭危险因素的积累进行风险评估是不现实的。许多危险因素不可改变。

对危险因素的认识可能会提醒临床医生注意一般的危险,但最重要的是关键的情境触发因素以及患者当前的精神状态、自杀意图和行为。

Basing the assessment of risk on an accumulation of risk factors alone is not realistic. Many risk factors are not modifiable. Awareness of the risk factors may alert the clinician to general levels of risk, but it is the key contextual triggering factors and the person's current mental state, suicide intent and behavior that are most immediately important.

最后,自杀风险水平的制定还应确定最适当的护理环境,以解决该风险并提供护理需求。在确定护理环境时,首先要考虑安全性,与能够维持自身安全的患者相比,被评估为有明确自杀意图的患者需要更高水平的安全保护。

Finally, the formulation of the level of risk for suicide should also determine the most appropriate care environment in which to address the risk and provide the care needed. The first priority in determining the care setting is safety. Patients assessed as having a clear intention of taking their lives will require higher levels of safety protection than those who are able to maintain their own safety.

(3)建立多轴诊断。

(3)Establish Multi-Axis Diagnosis.

研究表明,90%以上的自杀死亡者符合一种或多种精神疾病的标准。因此,临床医务工作者应该确定患者是否有轴Ⅰ或轴Ⅱ的诊断。自杀和其他自杀行为也更有可能发生在患有不止一种精神疾病的人身上。因此,需要注意当前或过去的Ⅰ轴或Ⅱ轴诊断,也包括那些当前可能处于缓解期的诊断。

Studies have shown that more than 90% of individuals who die by suicide satisfy the criteria for one or more psychiatric disorders. Thus, the clinicians should determine whether a patient has a primary axis Ⅰ or axis Ⅱ diagnosis. Suicide and other suicide behaviors are also more likely to occur in individuals with more than one psychiatric diagnosis. As a result, it is important to note other current or past axis Ⅰ or axis Ⅱ diagnoses, including those that may currently be in remission.

确定身体疾病(轴Ⅲ)是必不可少的,因为这种诊断也可能与自杀以及其他自杀行为的风险增加有关。对某些人来说,这种风险的增加可能是由于共病精神疾病的发病率增加、生理疾病或其治疗的直接生理影响造成的。身体疾病也可能是社会或心理压力的来源,这反过来也会增加自杀风险。

Identification of physical illness (axis Ⅲ) is essential since such diagnoses may also be associated with an increased risk of suicide as well as with an increased risk of other suicide behaviors. For some individuals, this increase in risk may result from increased rates of comorbid psychiatric illness or from the direct physiological effects of physical illness or its treatment. Physical illnesses may also be a source of social or psychological stress, which in turn may augment risk.

确定自杀风险的另一个关键因素是对心理社会应激源(轴Ⅳ)的识别,这些应激源可能是急性或慢性的。某些应激,如突然失业、人际关系丧失、社会孤立和人际关系失调,都会增加自杀未遂的可能性,并增加自杀的风险。

Also crucial in determining suicide risk is the recognition of psychosocial stressors (axis Ⅳ), which may be either acute or chronic. Certain stressors, such as sudden unemployment, interpersonal loss, social isolation, and dysfunctional relationships, can increase the likelihood of suicide attempts as well as increase the risk of suicide.

同时,重要的是要注意,生活事件对不同的个人有不同的意义。因此,在确定一个特定的压力源是否会带来自杀行为的风险时,有必要考虑对个体患者来说生命事件的重要性和意义。

At the same time, it is important to note that life events have different meanings for different individuals. Thus, in determining whether a particular stressor may confer risk for suicide behavior, it is necessary to consider the perceived importance and meaning of the life events for the individual patient.

作为多轴诊断的最后一个组成部分,评估患者的基线和当前的功能水平也非常重要(轴Ⅴ),同时,临床医生还应该评估患者功能水平的相对变化以及患者对其功能的看法和感受。虽然自杀意念或自杀未遂反映在整体功能评定量表(GAF)评分建议中,但应该指出,GAF 评分与自杀风险水平之间没有一致的相关性。

As the final component of the multiaxial diagnosis, the patient's baseline and current levels of functioning are important to assess (axis Ⅴ). Also, the clinician should assess the relative change in the patient's level of functioning and the patient's view of and feelings about his or her functioning. Although suicide ideation or suicide attempts are reflected in the Global Assessment of Functioning (GAF) scoring recommendations, it should be noted that there is no agreed-on correlation between a GAF score and level of suicide risk.

(4)自杀风险患者常见的精神症状。

(4)Common Psychiatric Symptoms in Patients at Risk of Suicide.

①焦虑。

①Anxiety.

焦虑似乎会增加自杀风险,尤其是严重的带有主观恐惧或忧虑的精神焦虑,不管这种感受是否有具体的焦虑对象。临床观察表明,焦虑患者可能比那些有抑郁症状包括精神运动抑制的个体更倾向于冲动自杀。

Anxiety appears to increase the risk for suicide. Specifically implicated has been severe psychic anxiety consisting of subjective feelings of fearfulness or apprehension, whether or not the feelings are focused on specific concerns. Clinical observation suggests that anxious patients may be more inclined to act on suicidal impulses than individuals whose depressive symptoms include psychomotor slowing.

对情感障碍患者自杀的研究表明,在患病后一年内自杀死亡的患者出现严重的心理焦虑或惊恐发作的可能性更大。在一个住院患者样本中,4/5 的患者在自杀前一周发生严重的焦虑、激动或两者兼有。

Studies of suicide in patients with affective disorders have shown that those who died by suicide within the first year after contact were more likely to have severe psychic anxiety or panic attacks. In an inpatient sample, severe anxiety, agitation, or both were found in four-fifths of patients in the week preceding suicide.

也有部分研究发现了焦虑与自杀未遂之间的类似联系,但不是所有的研究都是如此。由于严重的焦虑似乎确实会增加自杀风险,至少在某些患者群体中是这样,因此焦虑应该被视为自杀的一个经常被隐藏但可改变的危险因素。

Similar associations of anxiety with suicide attempts have been noted in some but not all studies. Since severe anxiety does seem to increase suicide risk, at least in some subgroups of patients, anxiety should be viewed as an often hidden but potentially modifiable risk factor for suicide.

②绝望。

②Hopelessness.

证据表明,绝望是一种与自杀风险增加相关的心理因素。绝望可能在程度上有所不同,从对未来的消极期望到对未来毫无希望甚至是绝望。一般来说,绝望程度高的患者未来自杀的风险更高。

Hopelessness is well established as a psychological dimension that is associated with increased suicide risk. Hopelessness may vary in degree from having a negative expectation for the future to being devoid of hope and despairing for the future. In general, patients with high levels of hopelessness have an increased risk for future suicide.

然而,在酒精使用障碍患者中,绝望的存在可能不会带来额外的风险。对于抑郁症患者,绝望被认为是解释为什么一些患者选择自杀,而另一些患者不选择自杀的因素。绝望还会导致自杀意念和自杀未遂的增加以及自杀意图强烈程度的增加。

However, among patients with alcohol use disorders, the presence of hopelessness may not confer additional risk. For patients with depression, hopelessness has been suggested to be the factor that explains why some patients choose suicide, whereas others do not. Hopelessness also contributes to an increased likelihood of suicide ideation and suicide attempts as well as an increased level of suicide intent.

作为一种"情境关联"的特征,绝望通常与抑郁症同时出现。但一些人在更主要、更持久的基础上经历了绝望。高基线水平的绝望也与自杀的可能性增加有关。

Hopelessness often occurs in concert with depression as a "state-dependent" characteristic, but some individuals experience hopelessness on a primary and more enduring basis. High baseline levels of hopelessness have also been associated with an increased likelihood of suicide behaviors.

然而,经历相似程度抑郁的患者可能有不同程度的绝望,而这种差异,反过来,可能会影响他们产生自杀想法的可能性。无论绝望的来源或主观概念是什么,减少绝望的干预措施可能会减少自杀的可能性。

However, patients experiencing similar levels of depression may have differing levels of hopelessness, and this difference, in turn, may affect their likelihood of developing suicide thoughts. Whatever the source or conceptualization of hopelessness, interventions that reduce hopelessness may be able to reduce the potential for suicide.

③冲动和攻击性。

③Impulsiveness and Aggression.

冲动与更高的自杀未遂率和更大的致死性有关(Javdani et al.,2011),并且通常与边缘型人格(LeGris J,2006)、双相情感障碍、酒精依赖有关,以及继发于严重抑郁的执行功能障碍(Keilp et al.,2001)。轻度至重度的颅脑外伤还与越来越多抑制解除/冲动增加有关,并与自杀行为增加有关(Yurgelun-Todd et al.,2011)。社会支持的增加可以减轻冲动(Kleiman et al.,2012)。

Impulsivity has been correlated with higher rates and greater lethality of suicide attempts, and is commonly associated with borderline personality, bipolar disorder, alcohol dependence, and executive dysfunction secondary to major depression. Mild to severe traumatic brain injuries are also associated with increased disinhibition/impulsivity and correlated with increased suicide behavior. Increased social support may mitigate impulsiveness.

矛盾的是,虽然对自杀的非专业和专业的看法都强调冲动的作用,但当前的研究表明,大多数自杀实际上是按照计划进行的,因此是可以预见的。这个区别的要点在于"冲动状态"(传统观念的自杀是冲动行为导致的)和贯穿人一生中表现出的"特质或人格变量"的冲动。

Paradoxically, while commonly held lay and even professional perceptions of suicide include the notion that most involve impulsivity, current research demonstrates that most suicides actually follow a plan, and thus are potentially foreseeable. This important distinction is based upon the critical difference between "state impulsivity" (traditional notion of suicide resulting from impulsive act) and impulsivity as a "trait or personality variable" exhibited throughout one's life.

这与基于研究的最新理解(托马斯·乔纳)相对应,该研究表明自杀涉及三个关键因素:认为自己对他人造成负担;缺乏归属感;一种从经历某些事件中增强的自杀能力和对于自杀的无畏感。随后的研究表明,冲动性格不能预测自杀未遂的冲动性,而非冲动性自杀未遂的杀伤力更强(Smith et al.,2008)。

This corresponds to recent understanding based on research (Thomas Joiner) indicating suicides involve 3 critical factors: a sense of perceiving oneself as burdensome to others; a lack of belonging; a learned capability for self-injury based upon experiencing activities that "foster fearlessness of and competence for suicide." Subsequent research has demonstrated that impulsive traits do not predict suicide attempt impulsivity, and that non-impulsive attempts are more lethal.

个人的冲动程度应作为自杀风险评估的一个组成部分,因为"冲动增加了个人获得自杀能力的可能性。"(Smith et al.,2008)此外,临床医生"不应过分关注个人本身的冲动水平;相反,应该花更多的时间来确定个人的冲动水平是否实际上导致了充满痛苦和挑衅性经历的生活方式,这也应包括在风险评估中。"

An individual's degree of impulsivity should be one component of the assessment of risk for suicide, as "impulsivity increases the likelihood that an individual will acquire the capability for suicide." Furthermore, clinicians "should not be overly focused on an individual's level of impulsivity per se; rather, more time should be spent determining whether the individual's level of impulsivity has in fact led to a lifestyle fraught with painful and provocative experiences, which should be included in the risk assessment as well".

冲动、敌意和攻击性可能单独或共同作用增加自杀风险。例如,许多研究为与冲动和敌意相关的影响和行为在自杀诊断中的作用提供了适度有力的证据。多项其他研究也表明,有自杀未遂史的人冲动和攻击的程度有所提高。许多边缘型人格障碍患者表现出自残行为,总的来说,这种行为与冲动增加有关。

Impulsivity, hostility, and aggression may act individually or together to increase suicide risk. For example, many studies provide moderately strong evidence for the roles of impulsivity and hostility-related affects and behavior in suicide across diagnostic groups. Multiple other studies have also demonstrated increased levels of impulsivity and aggression in individuals with a history of attempted suicide. Many patients with borderline personality disorder exhibit self-mutilating behaviors, and, overall, such behavior are associated with increased impulsivity.

然而,对于许多自残的患者来说,这些行为是有预谋的而不是冲动的。因此单独的自残行为不应被视为高度冲动的标志。此外,攻击性和冲动的评估并不是高度相关的,这也使得攻击性不能作为冲动的评估标准。因此,在精神检查和自杀风险评估中,冲动、敌意、攻击性和自残行为应该单独评估。

However, for many self-mutilating patients, these behaviors are premeditated rather than impulsive. Consequently, self-mutilation behaviors alone should not be regarded as an indicator of high impulsivity. Moreover, measures of aggression and impulsivity are not highly correlated, making aggression a poor marker of impulsivity as well. Thus, impulsivity, hostility, aggression, and self-mutilation behaviors should be considered independently in the psychiatric evaluation as well as in estimating suicide risk.

(5)患者自杀危险因素与警示信号。

(5)Risk Factors and Warning Signs of Suicide in Patients.

即使在没有明确自杀倾向的情况下,护士对危险因素的了解也可能有助于识别有自杀意念和行为的人。危险因素包括那些在大量人群中被研究并被证明与自杀可能性增加有关的特征。

Even in the absence of expressed suicidality, the nurse's knowledge of risk factors may help to identify individuals with suicide ideation and behaviour. Risk factors include those characteristics that have been studied in large populations and have been shown to be associated with an increased likelihood of suicide.

危险因素可分为动态因素和静态因素,也可分为可变因素和不可变因素。可变的危险因素是那些可以改变的因素。这一点很重要,因为可变危险因素的识别应该用于指导有关干预和支持计划的决策。可变危险因素包括抑郁、焦虑、绝望、药物使用、中毒和致命手段的获取。

Risk factors can be categorized as being either dynamic and modifiable or static and unmodifiable. Modifiable risk factors are those that are amendable to change. This is an important point, as the identification of modifiable risk factors should be used to direct decision-making regarding intervention and support planning (APA, 2003). Examples of modifiable risk factors include depression, anxiety, hopelessness, substance use, intoxication and access to lethal means.

相比之下,静态危险因素是那些无法改变的因素,如年龄、性别和自杀未遂史。尽管对危险因素的了解并不能让临床医生预测患者是否或何时会死于自杀,但对风险因素的识别是促进这些患者安全的一个重要组成部分。

In contrast, static risk factors are those that cannot be changed, such as age, gender and history of suicide attempts. Although knowledge of risk factors does not permit the clinician to predict if or when a client will die by suicide, the recognition of risk is a major component of promoting the safety of these clients.

除了解危险因素之外,了解自杀的警示信号也很重要。虽然危险因素已被证明是与自杀可能性增加有关的特征,但警示信号可能是提醒护士注意当前危险的明显迹象或症状。

In addition to knowledge of risk factors, it is important to be aware of warning signs for suicide. Whereas risk factors are characteristics that have been shown to be associated with an increased likelihood of suicide, warning signs may be overt signs or symptoms that alert the nurse to a current risk.

警示信号如下(患者和/或其家人、朋友、社区支持人员、医疗记录和精神卫生专业人员可报告或观察以下信息):

Warning Signs (The following information may be reported or observed by the client and/or their family, friends, community supporters, medical records and mental health professionals):

• 直接谈论自杀或死亡(如"我希望我已经死了");
• 间接谈论自杀或死亡,包括绝望和无价值的主题(如"继续下去有什么意义?""我累了""没有我,每个人都会过得更好");
• 威胁自杀,描述自杀的方法或在网上研究自杀的方法;
• 制定自杀计划;
• 自杀意念强度增加;
• 安排后事(如写下或修改遗嘱、捐赠钱或财物、把遗体捐献给科学、道别、写自杀遗书);

- 购买或储存药物、火器、剃须刀；
- 寻找阳台、桥梁、屋顶；
- 从事危险行为(如增加酒精或物质的使用、鲁莽驾驶)；
- 自我忽视(如外表的变化,包括体重和食欲的变化)；
- 性格改变；
- 情绪变化(如抑郁、焦虑、激动)；
- 社交退缩和孤立,包括在活动中失去享受。
- Talking about suicide or death directly (e.g., "I wish I was dead")；
- Talking about suicide or death indirectly, including themes of hopelessness and worthlessness (e.g., "What's the point of going on?" "I'm tired" "Everyone would be better off without me")；
- Threatening suicide, describing methods of suicide or researching methods of suicide on the Internet；
- Formation of suicide plans；
- Increased intensity of suicide ideation；
- Putting affairs in order (e.g., making or changing a will, giving money or possessions away, donating one's body to science, saying goodbye, writing suicide notes)；
- Purchasing or stockpiling medications, firearms, razors；
- Exploring balconies, bridges, rooftops；
- Engaging in risky behaviour (e.g., increased use of alcohol or substances, reckless driving)；
- Self-neglect (e.g., change in appearance, including changes in weight and appetite)；
- Change in personality；
- Change in mood (e.g., depression, anxiety, agitation)；
- Social withdrawal and isolation, including a loss of enjoyment in activities.

2.4 自杀风险患者的护理决策

2.4 Care Decisions for Suicidal Risk Patients

"认真对待"是指进行自杀风险评估,评估结果记录,与患者医疗团队的其他成员讨论评估结果,并根据评估结果制定安全和护理计划。

"Taking seriously" means to conduct a suicide risk assessment, to document the assessment, to discuss the assessment with other members of the client's health care team and create a plan for safety and care as determined by the outcome of the assessment.

2.4.1 决策支持工具

2.4.1 The Decision Support Tool

决策支持工具是基于专家共识开发的二级筛查工具,旨在帮助卫生服务提供者做出有关存在自杀风险的成年患者护理和出院的决策。它表明在简短干预后,门诊环境是否可以满足患者的健康和安全需求,或者是否首先需要心理健康专家对患者进行评估。

The decision support tool is a secondary screening instrument developed by expert consensus to help health service providers make decisions about the care and discharge of adult patients with suicide risk. It indicates whether a patient's health and safety needs are met in the outpatient environment following a brief intervention or whether evaluation from a mental health specialist may be needed first.

决策支持工具是为已被确定为具有自杀风险(即有自杀意念或怀疑自杀风险)且有能力做出医疗保健决策的成年患者设计使用的。这些患者的识别结果可通过下列资料产生:①患者披露;②家人、朋友、警察或其他相关人员的报告;③患者个人表现,如抑郁症、物质滥用或衰弱性疾病等;④初步自杀风险筛查。该决策支持工具不能替代卫生服务提供者的最佳判断或经验。

The decision support tool is designed for use with adult patients who have been identified as having suicide risk (i.e., suicide ideation or suspected suicide risk) and who have the capacity to make health care decisions. Identification of these patients may occur as a result of ① patient disclosure; ② reports by family, friends, police, or other collaterals; ③ individual patient presentations, such as depression, substance use, or debilitating illness; ④ primary screening. The decision support tool does not replace a provider's best judgment or experience.

医疗机构的临床人员角色各不相同,不同层级医疗卫生保健单位医生、护士和心理健康专家均可以使用决策支持工具。

Clinical staffing roles vary in medical institutions, and the decision support tool may be used by physicians, nurses, and mental health specialists in medical and health care institutions at different levels。

决策支持工具是一种二级筛查工具,可以帮助卫生服务提供者做出临床实践决策,例如"我可以在未咨询心理健康专家的情况下做出患者的处置决定吗?"和"在提供简短的干预措施后让患者出院是否合适?"等决策问题。

The decision support tool is a secondary screening tool that helps providers with practical decisions, such as "Can I make a disposition decision without consulting a mental health specialist?" and "Is it appropriate to discharge this patient after providing a brief ED-based intervention?"

初级筛查工具用于检测每一位患者（普遍筛查）或那些自杀风险高于平均水平的患者群体（选择性筛查），例如存在抑郁症状的患者。初级筛查并不揭示可能存在的自杀风险的性质。

Primary screening tools are used to detect possible suicide risk in every patient (universal screening) or in patients belonging to groups shown to be at a higher-than-average risk of suicide (selective screening), such as patients with depression. Primary screening does not uncover the nature of suicide risk that may be present.

不同工具之间的关系

工具类型	适用对象	评估结果
初级筛查工具（普查或选择性筛查）	所有急诊科患者或已知危险因素的患者	是否存在自杀风险
二级筛查工具（决策支持工具）	通过普查、患者披露或其他指标确定具有自杀风险的患者	患者接受简要干预措施后出院是否合适或需要心理健康专家进一步评估才能做出处置决定
全面的自杀风险评估	决策支持工具评估出的阳性自杀风险患者	患者风险和保护因素信息、即时风险和治疗需求

注：如果资源允许，自杀风险评估可以用于任何有自杀风险的患者

The Relationships among These Different Tools

TYPES OF TOOLS	SUBJECTS	OUTCOMES
Primary Screening Tool (universal or selective)	Every ED patient or patients with known risk factors	Whether suicide risk is present or absent
Secondary Screening Tool (Decision Support Tool)	Patients with some suicide risk as identified through universal screening, patient disclosure, or other indicators	Whether discharge following ED-based interventions is appropriate or further assessment by a mental health specialist is needed to make a disposition determination

TYPES OF TOOLS	SUBJECTS	OUTCOMES
Comprehensive Suicide Risk Assessment	Patients with suicide risk who score positive on the decision support tool	Information about a patient's risk and protective factors, immediate danger, and treatment needs

Note: If resources permit, a suicide risk assessment may be used with any patient with suicide risk.

决策支持工具表明在急诊科就诊期间哪些有自杀风险的患者可能需要进行心理健康评估(其中应包括自杀风险评估)。关于患者入院的知情决策结合了全面的自杀风险评估结果、卫生服务提供者的临床判断、患者和他/她的社会支持者的意见、患者护理专业团队的意见,以及该机构关于患者自杀评估与管理的政策和程序。

The decision support tool indicates which patients with suicide risk may need a mental health evaluation (which should include a suicide risk assessment) during the ED visit. Informed decisions about admission combine the results of a comprehensive suicide risk assessment, the provider's clinical judgment, input from the patient and his or her social supporters, input from the team of professionals caring for the patient, and the institution's policies and procedures for suicide evaluation and management.

初级筛查、二次筛查和自杀风险评估是截然不同但相关的临床实践过程,旨在帮助卫生服务提供者了解患者自杀风险的性质。

Primary screening, secondary screening, and suicide risk assessment are distinct but related practices designed to help providers understand the nature of their patients' suicide risk.

决策支持工具是一个六项条目、以"是/否"作为反映选项的工具。没有编号的第一个条目是不计分的,旨在确认患者是否存在自杀风险并作为询问自杀相关主题的过渡选项。对编号为1到6的条目进行评分。该工具后面的内容是对其使用方法的分步说明。

The decision support tool is a six-item, "yes/no" response tool. The first item, with no number, is unscored and is designed to confirm that suicide risk exists and to transition into the topic of suicide. Items numbered 1 through 6 are scored. Step-by-step instructions follow the tool.

决策支持工具

	过渡问题:确认自杀意念 最近你有过自杀的想法吗？ 是否有其他显示患者存在自杀意念的证据,例如家人或朋友的报告?(不计分)	Y	
1	考虑自杀计划的实施:最近你是否考虑过如何结束自己的生命?	Y	N
2	自杀意图:你是否有任何结束自己生命的意图?	Y	N
3	自杀未遂史:你是否曾经试图结束自己的生命?	Y	N
4	重大心理健康状况:你是否接受过心理健康问题的治疗? 你现在有无影响自身生活能力的心理健康问题?	Y	N
5	物质使用障碍:您是否曾在过去一个月内使用酒精饮料的次数达到四次或更多(针对女性)/五次或更多(针对男性)? 或者您在过去一个月内因非医疗原因使用过毒品或药物吗? 使用酒精或毒品对你来说是个困扰吗?	Y	N
6	易怒/易激动/具有攻击性:最近你是否感到非常焦虑或容易激动? 你有没有参与到冲突或斗殴事件? 是否存在烦躁、易激动或具有攻击性的直接证据?	Y	N

Decision Support Tool

	Transition question：Confirm Suicide Ideation Have you had recent thoughts of killing yourself? Is there other evidence of suicide thoughts, such as reports from family or friends?(Not part of scoring)	Y	
1	Thoughts of carrying out a plan：Recently, have you been thinking about how you might kill yourself?	Y	N
2	Suicide intent：Do you have any intention of killing yourself?	Y	N
3	Past suicide attempt：Have you ever tried to kill yourself?	Y	N
4	Significant mental health condition：Have you had treatment for mental health problems? Do you have a mental health issue that affects your ability to do things in life?	Y	N

5	Substance use disorder: Have you had four or more (female) or five or more (male) drinks on one occasion in the past month or have you used drugs or medication for non-medical reasons in the past month? Has drinking or drug use been a problem for you?	Y	N
6	Irritability/agitation/aggression: Recently, have you been feeling very anxious or agitated? Have you been having conflicts or getting into fights? Is there direct evidence of irritability, agitation, or aggression?	Y	N

决策支持工具的使用

Usage of the Decision Support Tool

第一步：告知患者。

告知您的患者，您将询问几个问题，以帮助您考虑后续护理计划与决策。

STEP 1: Inform the patient.

Tell your patient that you will be asking a few questions to help you consider next steps.

第二步：回顾患者的自杀意念。

如果这是您与患者的第一次沟通，首先要确认他/她是否有自杀意念。直接询问患者或陈述您对患者自杀风险性质的理解，这个过程将有助于卫生服务提供者顺利过渡到第1个条目（即计划）。

STEP 2: Review the patient's suicide ideation.

If this is your first interaction with the patient, begin by confirming that he or she has suicide ideation. Ask the patient directly or state your understanding of the nature of his or her suicide risk. This will facilitate a smooth transition to item number 1 (plan).

第三步：依次询问条目 1—6。

该工具包含关于如何进行询问的示例。根据开放的、非判断性的原则来克服社会反应偏见并鼓励患者真实地回答。

STEP 3: Ask questions for items 1 through 6.

The tool includes example questions to ask. Use an open, nonjudgmental style to overcome social response bias and encourage honest answers.

第四步：回顾其他可获得信息。

使用可获得数据（例如，患者观察报告或医疗记录），并咨询相关人员（例如，朋友、家庭成员和门诊卫生服务提供者)以证实患者的报告。让患者知道您可能联系他/她的相关人员,并且在您等待证明信息的同时可能会延缓急诊科就诊过程。

STEP 4: Review other available information.

Use available data (e.g., patient observations, medical records) and consult with available collaterals (e.g., friends, family members, and outpatient providers) to corroborate the patient's report. Let the patient know you would like to contact his or her collaterals, and that the visit may be delayed while you are awaiting corroborating information.

卫生服务提供者可以与他人分享患者健康信息吗?

可以。针对考虑存在自杀风险且最小化或否认自身自杀风险的患者,联系她/他的相关人员以获得真实信息是可能挽救生命的。首先征求患者允许与其朋友、家人或门诊治疗提供者取得联系的许可。如果在合理怀疑患者存在自杀未遂的前提下患者仍然拒绝授予联系权,则在未经患者许可的情况下,卫生服务提供者有权利联系患者的相关人员。

Can health service providers share patient health information with others?

Yes. For patients with concerning risk factors who minimize or deny suicide risk, it may be life-saving to contact collaterals for corroborating information. First request the patient's permission to contact his/her friends, family, or outpatient treatment providers. If the patient declines to consent after reasonable attempts have been made to obtain permission, there are circumstances in which collaterals may be contacted without the patient's permission.

第五步:核实分数。

每一项"是"的回答记为1分。条目1—6回答"是"的总次数即为患者总得分。

得分=0:如果对每个条目(1—6)的回答均为"否",则在提供一个或多个简要自杀预防干预措施后,允许患者出院可能是一个较为合适的护理决策。

得分≥1:如果对过渡问题(即自杀意念)并且条目1—6中任意一项的回答为"是",请考虑在就诊期间咨询心理健康专家以展开进一步评估,包括全面的自杀风险评估。

在确定后续护理计划时,请考虑患者即时的安全需求。如果评估结果将出院作为推荐的处置方式,请提供简要的自杀预防干预措施。

STEP 5: Check the score.

A "yes" response is equal to 1. Total the number of "yes" responses on items 1—6.

Score＝0. If the response to every item（1－6）is "no", discharge may be appropriate following the provision of one or more brief suicide prevention interventions.

Score≥1. If the responses to the transition question（i.e., suicide ideation）and any item 1－6 are "yes," consider consulting a mental health specialist during the visit for further evaluation, including a comprehensive suicide risk assessment.

Consider the immediate safety needs of the patient as you determine next steps. If the evaluation points to discharge as the recommended disposition, provide the brief suicide prevention interventions.

第六步：告知患者后续的护理决策。

向患者解释下一步的护理计划。例如：

得分＝0：假设您正在考虑将他/她送到门诊治疗机构，并打算先实施简单的干预措施，请向患者阐述您计划使用的干预措施，询问患者对此计划的反馈，并讨论他/她可能对此计划存在的任何保留意见。

得分≥1：假设您希望他/她在就诊时与专家见面，以便进一步评估病情。向患者解释，心理健康专家可能会重复您已经问过的问题。您要熟悉心理健康专家在评估中使用的自杀风险评估工具。

STEP 6：Tell the patient what happens next.

Explain next steps, for example：

Score＝0. Say that you are considering discharging him or her to an outpatient care setting and would first like to provide a brief intervention. Describe the intervention you plan to use. Ask for the patient's feedback on this plan and discuss any reservations he or she may have about it.

Score ≥1. Say that you would like him or her to see a specialist for further evaluation as part of the visit. Explain that the specialist may repeat some of the questions that you have already asked. Be familiar with the type of suicide risk assessment used in the mental health specialist's evaluation.

让患者参与决策过程。研究表明,共同决策过程可以降低患者压力,让患者产生控制感,并产生更好的结果。有自杀风险的患者在参与他们的护理决策时会表现出更高的满意度。

Involve the patient in the decision-making process. Research suggests that shared decision-making lowers patient stress, gives patients a sense of control, and leads to better outcomes. Patients with suicide risk report higher satisfaction when they are involved in decisions about their care.

提供一个估计的等待时间。如果等待时间过长,请询问什么能增加患者的舒适度。

Provide a waiting time estimate. If the waiting time is significant, ask what will increase the patient's comfort.

2.4.2 调动资源
2.4.2 Mobilize Resources

调动资源的目标是稳定当前的风险,并对持续风险进行症状管理。看似轻微的自残后遗症可能仍然与极度的情绪困扰有关,患者可能仍处于高风险状态,需要在适当的设施中进行全面彻底的评估。

The goal of mobilizing resources is stabilization of the immediate risk and symptom management for the ongoing risk. Seemingly minor sequelae of self-harm may still be associated with extreme emotional distress and the client may remain at a high risk and require a thorough holistic assessment in an appropriate facility.

一份安全计划是根据患者的情况来制定的,以自我监测绝望、无助和焦虑的感觉。制定一个结构化的安全计划包括消除自杀方法、调节情绪(缓解紧张)、提高症状管理基本技能等。安全计划还包括由护士或其他合格人员照顾患者,直至实施治疗计划。

A safety plan is developed with the input of the client to self-monitor feelings of hopelessness, helplessness and dysphoria. A structured plan to diffuse suicide methods, regulate emotions (reducing tension), develop basic skills of symptom management is developed. The safety plan includes attendance of the client by the nurse or other qualified personnel until a treatment plan is in place.

在某些情况下,获得小组或其他保健或紧急支持人员的帮助可能有限或不可行。在这种情况下,护士的首要任务是维护患者和其他人的安全,其主要目的是识别处于情绪痛苦状态的患者以及有自我伤害风险的患者,以创造一个安全的环境,并根据痛苦和自杀风险的严重程度来决定采取适当的行动。

In some situations, access to a team or other health care or emergency support personnel may be limited or not feasible. In such a situation, the nurse's priority is to maintain safety for the client and others. The main goal is to identify the client in a state of emotional distress and who is at risk of harming himself/herself, to create a safe environment and to take appropriate action determined by the severity of the distress and risk for suicide.

调动资源经常需要团队计划和支持。这可能包括以下行动:

• 确定关键的家庭成员、朋友、宗教团体成员,可从他们那里获得现场或电话支持(Holkup，2002)；

• 提高家人和朋友对情绪困扰和自杀风险的认知；

• 确定紧急服务，例如紧急医疗服务、危机应对服务、移动响应和在护士执业领域提供的诊所等(Holkup，2002)；

• 获得紧急或急迫的精神卫生服务（National Collaborating Centre for Mental Health，2004）；

• 寻找住院的替代方案；

• 与教牧、精神和其他咨询服务机构建立联系。

Mobilizing resources frequently requires a team plan and response. This may include actions such as:

• Identification of key family members, friends, members of a religious community, who can be available for on-site or telephone support;

• Improving the awareness of family and friends about emotional distress and risk of suicide;

• Identification of emergency services, such as emergency medical services, crisis response services, mobile response and walk-in clinics available in the nurses' area of practice;

• Accessing emergent or urgent mental health services;

• Finding alternatives to hospitalization;

• Connecting with pastoral, spiritual and other counseling services.

调动资源的注意事项：

• 护士评估风险等级；

• 护士根据评估的风险等级确定出紧急、急迫或选择性的资源；

• 护士调动适当的资源(正式和非正式)；

• 如果风险迫在眉睫，护士可直接调动适当的资源；

• 护士确保由合格人员来运送被监督的患者；

• 在发生自残或自杀未遂的情况下，调动资源是为了进行心理和体格评估。

Consideratons for mobilizing resources:

• The nurse assessing the level of risk;

• The nurse identifying emergent, urgent or elective resources based upon that assessed risk level;

• The nurse mobilying appropriate resources (formal and informal);

• The nurse mobilying appropriate resources directly if the risk is imminent;

• The nurse ensuring supervised client transported by qualified personnel;

• In the cases of self-harm or suicide attempt, the mobilization of resources being for both psychological and physical assessment.

2.4.3 观察等级和治疗环境的确定

2.4.3 Determination of Observation Level and Determination of Treatment Environment

立即对任何被认定为有自杀风险的个体进行观察。一旦完成全面评估,应根据需要调整支持和观察等级。在国际文献和指南中,特别是关于不同观察级别的特征以及可以启动或改变观测等级的条件,在实践中存在显著差异。

Observation begins immediately for anyone identified with suicide risk. Once a comprehensive assessment is completed, the level of support and observation should be adapted as required. In the international literature and guidelines, particularly with regard to the characteristics of different levels of observation and the conditions under which levels of observation can be initiated or changed, there are significant differences in practice.

因此,观察的目的是针对缺乏控制自杀意念能力的患者提供支持。本书建议,监测等级应反映患者变化的风险水平,这取决于临床判断和与卫生保健小组的协作。

Where by the purpose of observation is to provide support to clients who lack the capacity to prevent acting on suicide ideation. This book recommends that the level of monitoring reflect the client's changing level of risk, as determined by clinical judgment and collaboration with the health care team.

患者对了解和控制自伤行为的信心是决定最适当观察等级的一个重要因素。有关观察等级的决策还应考虑自杀风险水平、现有的监测支持、提供观察者的技能水平、环境和组织政策的适宜性。

The client's confidence of understanding and controlling self-harm behaviour is an important factor for determining the most appropriate observation level. Decisions about levels of observation should also involve a consideration of the level of suicide risk, existing supports for monitoring, the skill level of individuals providing observation, the suitability of the environment and organizational policies.

治疗环境,包括护士与患者之间的互动,这与被观察的患者体验密切相关。在对精神科住院患者的描述性研究中,琼斯和他的同事(2000)报告指出,当观察患者的护士对患者很熟悉,并且与其沟通交流而不是保持冷漠和沉默,许多患者会感到更安全、放心和关心,而不是被人打扰,并且感受到的挫折感更少。由于护士的态度和行为对患者体验的影响,作者建议观察应被视为是与患者进行治疗互动的机会。

The therapeutic milieu, including the nurse-client interaction, is closely tied to the experience of the client under observation. In their descriptive study of psychiatric inpatients, Jones and colleagues (2000) reported that when a nurse observing a patient was familiar with the patient and communicated with the patient rather than remaining cold and silent, many patients felt safer, more secure, and more concerned than disturbed, and experienced less frustration. Because of this influence of nurses' attitudes and behaviours on clients' experiences, the authors suggest that observation should be regarded as an opportunity to engage in therapeutic interactions with clients.

为有自杀或自杀行为风险的患者选择治疗环境的指南

(1) 住院治疗。

在自杀未遂的情况下:

• 患者有精神症状;

• 自杀未遂是暴力的、近乎致命的或有预谋的;

• 采取了预防措施以避免被救援或被发现;

• 存在持久性自杀计划或意图;

• 痛苦增加或患者后悔幸存;

• 患者为男性,年龄45岁以上,特别是有精神疾病或自杀想法的新发患者;

• 患者的家庭或社会支持有限,包括缺乏稳定的生活环境;

• 目前有冲动行为、十分激动、判断力下降或拒绝帮助;

• 患者的精神状态发生变化,其代谢、毒性、传染性或其他病因需要在结构化环境中进行进一步检查。

在有自杀意念的情况下:

• 具有高致命性的具体计划;

• 强烈的自杀意图。

Guidelines for Selecting a Treatment Setting for Patients at Risk for Suicide or Suicide Behaviors

(1) Admission Generally Indicated.

After a suicide attempt:

- The patient being psychotic;

- The attempt being violent, near-lethal, or premeditated;

- Precautions being taken to avoid rescue or discovery;

- The persistent plan or intent being present;

- Distress being increased or the patient regrets surviving;

- The patient being male, older than age 45 years, especially with new on-set of psychiatric illness or suicidal thinking;

- The patient having limited family and/or social support, including lack of stable living situation;

- Current impulsive behavior, severe agitation, poor judgment, or refusal of help being evident;

- The patient having changes in mental status with a metabolic, toxic, infectious, or other etiology requiring further workup in a structured setting.

In the presence of suicide ideation with:

- A specific plan with high lethality;

- A high suicide intent.

(2)可能需要住院治疗。

在自杀未遂后,一般要求住院治疗。

自杀意念通常由以下原因产生:

- 精神病性障碍;

- 重症精神障碍;

- 自杀未遂,特别是造成了严重的医学后果;

- 可能造成身体不良状况的原因(如急性神经障碍、癌症、感染);

- 对部分医院或门诊治疗缺乏反应或无法合作;

- 需要特定医疗条件的药物治疗或ECT;

- 需要临床观察、临床测验或诊断评估的配套设置;

- 有限的家庭或社会支持,包括生活状况缺乏稳定性;

- 目前没有稳定的治疗关系,或者医护人员无法定期随访。

(2)Admission May be Necessary.

After a suicide attempt, admission is generally indicated.

Suicide ideation generally resulting from:

• Psychosis;

• Major psychiatric disorder;

• Past attempts, particularly if medically serious;

• Possibly contributing medical condition (e.g., acute neurological disorder, cancer, infection);

• Lack of response or ability to cooperate with partial hospital or outpatient treatment;

• Need for supervised setting for medication trial or ECT;

• Need for skilled observation, clinical tests, or diagnostic assessments that require a structured setting;

• Limited family and/or social support, including lack of stable living situation;

• Lack of an ongoing clinician-patient relationship or lack of access to timely outpatient follow-up.

（3）门诊治疗。

如果没有自杀未遂或没有自杀意念/计划/意图,但是从精神病学评估或其他知情人提供的证据表明自杀风险很高,并且近期风险急剧增加,可能会结束急诊科治疗和并提供随访建议。

在自杀未遂或有自杀意念/计划的情况下:

•计划/方法和意图的致死率低;

•患者有稳定和支持的生活状况;

•患者能够配合建议进行随访。

（3）Outpatient Service.

In the absence of suicide attempts or reported suicide ideation/plan/intent, evidence from the psychiatric evaluation and/or history from others suggests a high level of suicide risk and a recent acute increase in risk. Release from emergency department with follow-up recommendations may be possible.

After a suicide attempt or in the presence of suicide ideation/plan when:

• The plan/method and intent having low lethality;

• The patient having stable and supportive living situation;

- The patient being able to cooperate with recommendations for follow-up.

（4）门诊治疗可能比住院治疗更有益。

患者有慢性自杀意念或自伤行为，但之前没有造成严重医疗后果；如果患者有安全和支持性的生活环境，并且正接受门诊精神专科治疗，可选择门诊治疗。

（4）Outpatient Treatment May be More Beneficial than Hospitalization.

The patient has chronic suicide ideation and/or self-injury without prior medically serious attempts, if a safe and supportive living situation is available and outpatient psychiatric care is ongoing.

小品文

Vignette

情景：上夜班时，注册护士为 60 岁的退休鳏夫癌症患者史密斯先生提供睡前药物时，患者叹了口气说："这一切都没有意义，像这样活下去太不值得，我现在应该安排后事了。"

Scenario：On the evening shift, the RN gives Mr. Smith, a 60-year-old retired widower with cancer, his bedtime medications. He sighs and says, "There is no point to any of this. It is not worth living like this. I should just get my affairs in order now."

护士反思：这位护士意识到，丧失亲人、抑郁和患病会使人有自杀意念和行为的风险。一系列的因素可能会使这位患者有自杀想法或行为的危险。虽然他并没有公开声明他想要自杀，但护士指出了间接的语言暗示和深深叹息的非言语暗示可能表示绝望。同时护士知道患者的心理社会背景也会增加他的自杀风险。

Nurse's Reflection：The nurse is aware that losses of relatives, a depressed state and a medical illness can put one at risk for suicide ideation and behaviour. The client has a constellation of factors when combined could put him at risk for suicide ideation and/or behaviour. Although he does not overtly state that he wants to take his life, the nurse identifies the indirect verbal cues and the non-verbal cue of deep sighing, which could indicate despair. The nurse is aware of the client's psychosocial background that also can increase his risk.

护士反应：护士认真对待患者的陈述，并进行自杀风险评估。

Nurse's Response：The nurse appropriately takes the client's statements seriously and conducts a suicide risk assessment.

---

3 患者自杀预防与干预

3 Suicide Prevention and Intervention in Patients

世界卫生组织(WHO)鼓励各国继续落实已经开展的有效的自杀预防工作，并将自杀预防置于工作议程的重中之重。自杀是可以通过采用及时有效的循证干预、治疗和支持预防的。

The World Health Organization (WHO) has said "preventing suicide, a global imperative", which encouraged countries to continue to implement effective suicide prevention efforts and to place suicide prevention at the top of their agenda. Suicide can be prevented with timely and effective evidence-based interventions, treatment and support.

自杀问题不仅给卫生部门带来负担，还给许多部门乃至整个社会都带来多重的不良影响。因此，要开启自杀预防工作的成功之旅，国家就应该将不同部门和相关利益方整合在一起，采取多部门协作的综合方式去解决自杀问题。

Suicide is not only a burden on the health sector, but also has multiple negative effects on many sectors and society as a whole. Therefore, to start a successful journey of suicide prevention, countries should integrate different departments and relevant stakeholders, and adopt a comprehensive approach of multi-department cooperation to solve the suicide problem.

在WHO《2013—2020年精神卫生行动计划》中，会员国承诺努力实现到2020年各国自杀率降低10％的全球目标。WHO于2008年启动的精神卫生差距行动计划将自杀作为优先条件之一，并提供循证技术指导，以扩大各国的服务提供。

In the WHO's Mental Health Action Plan 2013-2020, member states have committed themselves to work towards the global target of reducing the suicide rate in countries by 10％ in 2020. The WHO's Mental Health Gap Action Program, which was launched in 2008, regards suicide as one of the priority conditions and provides evidence-based technical guidance to expand service provision in countries.

美国自杀预防资源中心(SPRC)倡导指出："我们都应各尽其职。团结起来，我们就能拯救生命。"定性调查和临床经验表明，自杀是可以预防的，自杀风险也是可以降低的，在个人、社区和国家层面上可以采取很多措施来预防和减少自杀。

Suicide Prevention Resource Centre(SPRC) has advocated that"We all have a role to play. Together, we can save lives."It is clear from qualitative investigations and clinical expertise that suicide is preventable and the risk of suicide can be reduced, and much can be done to prevent and reduce suicide at individual, community and national levels.

目前,已出版了许多关于降低和预防自杀意念和自杀行为风险的指南,促进对个人和家庭的保护,完善患者生存理由,以及提供能够降低自杀风险的成功护理干预措施。截至2014年,已有28个国家建立了国家自杀预防策略。每年9月10日的世界预防自杀日,是由国际自杀预防协会组织的全球性自杀预防活动日。

Many guidelines have been published on reducing and preventing suicidal ideation and behavioral risk, promoting protection for individuals and families, improving reasons for survival, and providing successful nursing interventions that will reduce the risk of suicide. By 2014, 28 countries had established national suicide prevention strategies. World Suicide Prevention Day, organized by the international association for suicide prevention, is observed worldwide on September 10.

基于循证的自杀预防干预措施是在一个理论框架中组织起来的,该框架区分了普遍性的、选择性的和有针对性的干预措施。在实际应用中,干预措施的选择应根据实际情况而定,可不拘泥于该理论框架。干预措施可包含三种。

Evidence-based interventions for suicide prevention are organized in a theoretical framework that distinguishes between universal, selective and indicated interventions. These linkages are not finite, and in reality should be context-driven. The interventions include three kinds.

①普遍性预防策略旨在惠及全体人口,通过提供更多的护理和帮助,加强社会支持和改变物质环境等保护措施,以最大限度地提高健康水平和降低自杀风险。

①Universal prevention strategies are designed to reach an entire population in an effort to maximize health and minimize suicide risk by removing barriers to care and increasing access to help, strengthening protective processes such as social support, and altering the physical environment.

②选择性预防策略指根据年龄、性别、职业地位或家族史等特征,针对人口中的高危人群进行自杀预防。虽然部分个体目前可能没有表现出自杀行为,但他们可能具有较高的与自杀风险相关的生物学、心理学或社会经济学等特征。

②Selective prevention strategies target vulnerable groups within a population based on characteristics such as age, sex, occupational status or family history. While individuals may not currently express suicidal behaviors, but they may have higher biological, psychological, or socioeconomic characteristics associated with suicide risk.

③针对性预防策略指针对人群中特定的高危人群,例如那些表现出早期自杀倾向的人或自杀未遂的人。考虑到多种因素和多种途径可导致自杀行为,自杀预防工作需要多部门广泛协作,以期降低不同人群和不同风险组别全生命周期的自杀风险。

③ Indicated prevention strategies target specific vulnerable individuals within the population, e.g., those displayed early signs of suicide potential or who have made a suicide attempt. Given the multiple factors involved and the many pathways leading to suicidal behavior, suicide prevention requires a broad multidisciplinary approach that addresses the various population and risk groups and contexts throughout the life course.

与相关干预措施对应的关键自杀危险因素如下图3.1所示(线条反映的是针对不同危险因素的各层面干预措施的相对重要性):

Key risk factors for suicide are aligned with relevant interventions as shown in Figure 3.1:(Lines reflect the relative importance of interventions at different levels for different areas of risk factors)

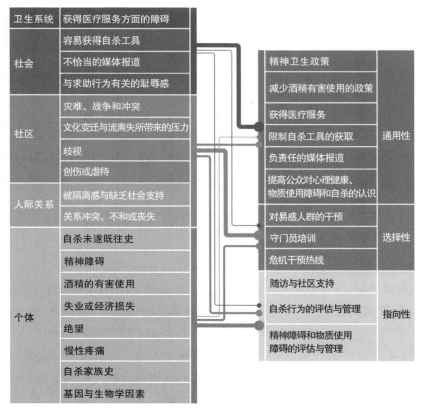

图3.1 关键自杀危险因素

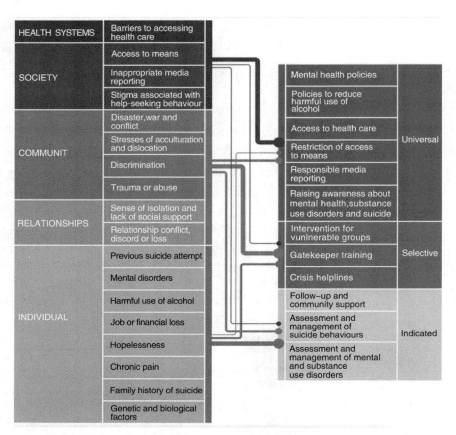

Figure 3.1　Key Risk Factors For Suicide

　　在本文中,我们重点介绍患者自杀预防与干预措施(针对性的干预措施)。针对有自杀意念、计划或行为的患者,自杀预防和干预包括一系列广泛的治疗干预,主要包括确立一个治疗和监督的环境,关注患者的安全,努力建立合作性和协作性的医患关系等。

　　In this book, we focus on suicide prevention and intervention measures in patients (indicated prevention strategies). Suicide prevention and intervention consist of a broad array of therapeutic interventions that should be instituted for patients with suicidal thoughts, plans, or behaviors. It majorly includes determining a setting for treatment and supervision, attending to patient safety, and working to establish a cooperative and collaborative physician-patient relationship, and so on.

　　对于正在接受治疗的患者,预防和干预也包括建立和维持治疗关系;不同临床医务工作者协作提供的治疗;监测患者的进展和对治疗计划的反应,并对患者的人身安全、精神状态和功能水平进行持续评估。此外,还可以包括鼓励患者坚持治疗和对患者进行教育,必要时,还可以对家属和其他重要人员提供健康教育。

For patients in ongoing treatment, prevention and intervention also include establishing and maintaining a therapeutic alliance; coordinating treatment provided by multiple clinicians; monitoring the patient's progress and response to the treatment plan; and conducting ongoing assessments of the patient's safety, psychiatric status, and level of functioning. Additionally, they may include encouraging treatment adherence and providing education to the patient. If necessary, health education can also be provided to family members and other important personnel.

3.1 建立和维持治疗关系

3.1 Establish and Maintain a Therapeutic Alliance

3.1.1 与患者建立治疗关系

3.1.1 Establish Treatment Alliances with Patients

治疗关系是指起始于护士和患者之间的人际关系,其具有目的性并旨在促进患者利益和治疗成效的最大化。影响治疗关系的因素包括积极倾听、信任、尊重、真诚、同情和对患者担忧的回应。

The therapeutic relationship describes an interpersonal process that occurs between the nurse and the client(s), which is purposeful and directed at advancing the client's best interest and outcomes. Factors influencing the therapeutic relationship include active listening, trust, respect, genuineness, empathy and responding to client concerns.

由于建立治疗关系涉及对伴有自杀意念或自杀行为风险患者的护理,它被认为是自杀预防的临床护理工作中必不可少的环节。治疗关系的确立有利于护理人员建立有益的治疗环境,在该环境中护理人员可以和患者高效地沟通并制定降低自杀预防策略。此外,有效的治疗和安全的治疗环境也能让患者感受到被尊重以及对其主观能动性的认可。

As it relates to the care of clients at risk for suicidal ideation or behavior, the establishment of a therapeutic relationship is considered essential for creating a context within which the nurse can actively engage with the client and develop strategies to reduce suicide risk. Furthermore, effective treatment and a safe treatment environment also allow patients to feel respected and recognized for their subjective initiative.

在帮助他们管理自己行为的同时,为其提供安全并维护他们的尊严。治疗性关系本身也可能治愈患者,因为它增强了希望,让患者感到被倾听、被尊重、被关怀。APA(2003)和 NZGG(2003)指南都表明积极的治疗性关系对自杀有保护作用。

It is about providing safety and maintaining their dignity, while assisting them in managing their behavior. As such, the therapeutic relationship may also be healing in itself, as it may foster a sense of hope while making patients feel heard, respected and connected. Both APA (2003) and NZGG (2003) guidelines suggest that positive therapeutic relationships have protective effects for suicide.

从最初与患者的接触开始,医护人员应该尝试与患者建立信任和相互尊重的治疗关系。可以在这种医患合作关系的背景下探索和确定患者的自杀意念和自杀行为,最终达到降低自杀风险的目标。

Beginning with the initial encounter with the patient, the medical staff should attempt to build trust, establish mutual respect, and develop a therapeutic relationship with the patient. Suicidal ideation and behaviors can be explored and addressed within the context of this cooperative doctor-patient relationship, with the ultimate goal of reducing suicide risk.

这种关系还提供了可以评估和治疗其他精神症状或综合征的环境。与此同时,医护人员应该认识到,一个决心自杀的人可能并不想发展医患合作的关系,实际上可能会将精神科医师视为敌人。

This relationship also provides a context in which additional psychiatric symptoms or syndromes can be evaluated and treated. At the same time, the medical staff should recognize that an individual who is determined to die may not be motivated to develop a cooperative doctor-patient relationship and indeed may view the psychiatrist as an adversary.

深入了解患者重要的人际关系,可以帮助医护人员了解患者是否愿意建立牢固的治疗关系。此外,通过密切关注患者及其家属对治疗的期望可以增强治疗关系。

An in-depth understanding of the patient's important relationships can help healthcare professionals understand whether the patient is willing to suggest a strong therapeutic relationship. In addition, the therapeutic alliance can be enhanced by paying careful attention to the concerns of patients and their family members as well as their wishes for treatment.

对自杀患者的同情心和理解有利于帮助患者建立治疗性的医患关系,帮助患者感受情感支持,以及认识除了自杀还存在其他的选择。如此,积极合作的治疗关系就显得尤为宝贵,甚至可能成为自杀患者赖以生存的力量来源。

Empathy and understanding of the suicidal individual are also important in establishing a therapeutic medical staff-patient relationship, helping the patient feel emotionally supported, and increasing the patient's sense of possible choices other than suicide. In this manner, a positive and cooperative therapeutic relationship can be an invaluable and even life-sustaining force for suicidal patients.

在照顾有潜在自杀倾向的患者时,医护人员需要处理好相互矛盾的目标,既要鼓励患者的独立性,又要兼顾安全性。此外,医护人员应该意识到自己对自杀患者的情绪和反应可能会影响患者的治疗。

In caring for potentially suicidal patients, the medical staff need to manage the often competing goals of encouraging the patient's independence yet simultaneously addressing safety. In addition, the medical staff should be aware of his or her own emotions and reactions to the suicidal patient in case they have an effect on the patient's treatment.

医护人员应该认识到他们可能在患者生活中所处的独特地位,因为他们通常会被患者当作活下去的唯一理由。与此同时,医护人员必须防止陷入永久救世主的角色。有自杀倾向的患者可能希望得到无条件的照顾,也可能希望让其他人为他们继续活下去担责。

Medical staff should acknowledge the unique place that they may hold in a patient's life, often seeming to be the only source of stability or consistency. At the same time, the medical staff must guard against falling into the role of a constant savior. Suicidal patients may wish to be taken care of unconditionally or alternatively, to assign others the responsibility for keeping them alive.

那些被有自杀倾向的患者当作救世主的医护人员,通常会有意或无意地假设他们能够提供别人无法提供的爱和关怀,从而神奇地将患者的死亡愿望转变为对生存的渴望。

Therapists who are drawn into the role of a savior with suicidal patients often operate on the conscious or unconscious assumption that they can provide love and concern that others cannot provide, thus magically transforming the patient's wish to die into a desire to live.

如果出现这种情况,或者医护人员使用防御性反应来否定对患者的敌意,那么医务人员可能就需要花费大量时间向患者保证他或她对患者只有积极的感受,并且会采取一切必要措施来挽救患者的生命。在最糟糕的情况下,就需告知患者过度的个人关怀可能会影响甚至破坏治疗关系。

Under such circumstances, or if the therapist uses defensive reaction formation to deny hostile feelings toward the patient, the therapist may go to great lengths to assure the patient that he or she has only positive feelings about the patient and will do whatever necessary to save the patient's life. In the worst-case scenario, this need to demonstrate one's caring may contribute to boundary crossings or outright boundary violations.

此外,由于给予患者错误或不现实的希望,医护人员最终可能会因未能实现这些期望而使患者失望。因此,医护人员必须记住,对患者的治疗负责并不等同于对患者的生活负责。

Also, by producing false or unrealistic hopes, the medical staff may ultimately disappoint the patient by not fulfilling those expectations. Thus, the medical staff must remember that taking responsibility for a patient's care is not the same as taking responsibility for a patient's life.

有自杀倾向的患者也可以激活医护人员自己对死亡和自杀的潜在情绪,从而导致作为医护人员的一些防御反应。一方面,有可能发展出对自杀患者的反移情仇恨和愤怒,这可能表现为医护人员的拒绝行为。

Suicidal patients can also activate a medical staff's own latent emotions about death and suicide, leading to a number of defensive responses as a medical staff. On one hand, there is a potential to develop countertransference hate and anger at suicidal patients that may be manifested by rejecting behavior on the part of the medical staff.

另一个极端是,医护人员可能会回避那些让自己对自杀感到焦虑的患者。医护人员也可能高估患者的能力,对患者产生不切实际的过高的期望。相反,他们可能会被患者的绝望所包围,对治疗的进展和患者自我改善的能力感到沮丧。

At the other extreme, the medical staff may avoid patients who bring up his or her own anxieties surrounding suicide. Medical staff may also overestimate the patient's capabilities, creating unrealistic and overwhelming expectations for the patient. Conversely, they may be surrounded by the patient's sense of hopelessness, and become discouraged about the progress of treatment and the patient's capacity to improve.

因此,识别移情和反移情的问题在治疗关系的管理中显得尤为重要,无论是心理治疗中的理论性操作程序还是治疗过程中明确发现有该类问题。在这方面,邀请高级别有经验的同行进行督导可能会更有裨益,或者求助于自杀管理方面的专家。还有一点很重要,治疗的过程和形式可能受到患者和治疗者之间的性别和文化差异,以及患者和其他医护人员文化差异的影响。

Thus, management of the therapeutic alliance should include awareness of transference and countertransference issues, regardless of the theoretical approach used for psychotherapy and whether these issues are directly addressed in treatment. In this regard, the use of consultation with a senior colleague with experience and expertise in the management of suicidal patients may be helpful. It is also important to keep in mind that the course and conduct of treatment may be influenced by gender and cultural differences between patients and therapists as well as by cultural differences between patients and other aspects of the care delivery system.

3.1.2 与其他临床工作者进行协作性照护

3.1.2 Coordinate Care and Collaborate with Other Clinicians

为有自杀行为的患者提供最佳治疗通常需要一个包括多名精神卫生工作人员的多学科治疗团队。与综合程度较低的门诊环境相比,总体治疗计划的持续协调通常更容易在住院部或局部医院环境中实施。在任何治疗环境中,提高团队协作的策略包括:明确的角色定义、团队成员之间的定期沟通以及提前制定的应急预案。

Providing optimal treatment for patients with suicidal behavior frequently involves a multidisciplinary treatment team that includes several mental health professionals. While ongoing coordination of the overall treatment plan is generally easier to implement in inpatient or partial hospital settings as opposed to less integrated ambulatory settings, useful strategies for coordination in any treatment setting include clear role definitions, regular communication among team members, and advance planning for management of crises.

有必要向患者说明这些人员将参与他们的治疗,并概述每个人的具体角色。在这一方面,重要的是让患者明白,治疗团队成员将从多方面协助精神科医生,并提供可影响风险防范级别、是否出院、药物和治疗计划其他方面决策的临床信息。

It is also helpful to clarify with the patient that a number of individuals will be involved in his or her care and to outline the specific roles of each. In this regard, it is important for patients to understand that treatment team members assist the psychiatrist in many respects and may supply clinical information that will influence decisions about the level of precautions, readiness for discharge, medications, and other aspects of treatment planning.

许多患者还伴有躯体疾病,常常会就诊于多个医生。特别是患者的躯体疾病可能会影响患者的精神症状,在其治疗时,及时和患者的社区医生或者患者就诊过的其他专科医生了解情况有利于治疗方案的制定。

Many patients have ongoing medical illnesses for which they receive care from one or more physicians. Particularly for individuals whose medical disorders or treatments interface with their psychiatric symptoms or treatments, it is helpful to communicate with the patient's primary care physician as well as with any specialists who are actively involved in the patient's care.

在住院环境中,治疗团队通常由精神科医生、护士、社会工作者、心理治疗师和其他精神卫生工作者组成。团队通常由精神科医生担任团队领导者,在治疗团队中其他成员的协作下,精神科医生将对患者的治疗做出关键的决定。

In inpatient settings, the treatment team generally consists of a psychiatrist, nurses, social workers, psychologists, and other mental health workers, with the psychiatrist acting as the team leader. In this capacity, with input from the other members of the team, the psychiatrist will make the critical decisions regarding the patient's treatment.

这些决定包括但不限于患者的诊断、具体用药、风险防范级别、通行、出院和后续的治疗计划。考虑到其他治疗小组成员的观察在这些决策中的关键作用,精神科医生应鼓励团队成员之间充分共享患者的病史和临床特征等信息。

Such decisions include but are not limited to the patient's diagnosis, specific medications, level of precautions, passes, discharge, and follow-up treatment plan. Given the key roles of the observations from other members in such decisions, the psychiatrist should encourage open communication among the staff members regarding historical and clinical features of the patient.

在门诊环境中也可能有其他专业人员参与患者的治疗。在某些情况下,患者可能会被转介给针对某个单一症状的专家(例如,绝望的认知行为治疗或复发性自杀行为的辩证行为治疗)。

In an outpatient setting, there might also involved other professionals in the care of patients. In some instances, patients may be referred to individuals with expertise in symptom-specific treatments (e.g., cognitive behavior therapy for hopelessness or dialectical behavior therapy for recurrent suicidal behavior).

有时主治精神科医生可能主要负责精神药理学管理,而由另一名精神科医生或其他精神卫生专业人员进行心理治疗。患者就诊时,主治精神科医生需要关注患者对各种治疗的反应。

In other instances, the psychiatrist may be providing primarily psychopharmacologic management, with another psychiatrist or other mental health professional conducting the psychotherapy. During visits with the patient, it is important for the psychiatrist to review the patient's response to all aspects of the treatment.

此外,如果患者发生重大临床变化,精神科医生应与治疗师沟通并制定指导方针,以确定何时以及在何种条件下应联系治疗师和精神科医生。此外,如果精神科医生对治疗师有直接的监督责任,那么更应加强沟通,包括共同完成病历分析。

In addition, it is useful for the psychiatrist to communicate with the therapist and to establish guidelines as to when and under what conditions the therapist and the psychiatrist should be contacted in the event of a significant clinical change in the patient. Moreover, if the psychiatrist has direct supervisory responsibilities for the therapist, the level of communication should be increased and may include a chart review.

3.2 简要自杀预防和干预措施

3.2 Brief Suicide Prevention and Intervention Measures

3.2.1 简要患者教育

3.2.1 Brief Patient Education

简要的患者教育干预有助于患者了解自身病情和治疗方案,并可以增加患者和家属对后续治疗的依从性。由于有自杀风险的患者在出院后通常不会参加心理健康的随访,因此住院期间可能是向患者及其家属提供重要自杀预防信息的最佳或唯一机会。书面材料可以作为补充但不能取代医护人员和患者之间面对面、一对一的沟通。

The brief patient education intervention helps the patient understand his or her condition and treatment options and may facilitate patient and family adherence to the follow-up plan. As patients with suicide risk often do not attend follow-up mental health appointments after discharge, the hospitalization may be the best or only opportunity to provide these patients and their family members with important suicide prevention information. Written materials may complement, but not replace, direct, one-on-one communication between the provider and the patient.

实施步骤:

得到患者的许可。在干预计划中纳入患者家人、亲密朋友和/或具备资质的陪伴康复师。陪伴康复师具有丰富的生活阅历,经过专业培训并获得相关资质。

Action Steps:

Ask the patient for permission to include his or her family members, close friends, and/ or a certified peer specialist in the intervention. A peer specialist is a person with a wealth of experience who is trained and certified to provide services to others.

与患者讨论以下内容：

- 患者的当前状况；
- 危险和保护因素；
- 治疗类型和选择治疗方案；
- 药物和依从性；
- 物质使用；
- 家庭护理；
- 致命性自杀方式的限制措施；
- 随访方案的推荐；
- 病情恶化的状况（例如，自杀意念的频率增加、睡眠问题增加）以及如何处理这些状况（例如，请朋友或家人帮助保护您的安全、消除致命性自杀方式的获得途径）。

Discussing the Following：

- Patient's current condition；
- Risk and protective factors；
- Type of treatment and options；
- Medications and adherence；
- Substance use；
- Home care；
- Lethal means restriction；
- Follow-up recommendations；
- Signs of a worsening condition (e.g., increased frequency of suicidal ideation, increased trouble sleeping) and how to respond (e.g., asking friends or family to help keep you safe, removing access to lethal means).

向患者传达治疗是有效的理念。例如，告诉患者"研究表明，心理健康治疗可以帮助人们从自杀的想法或感受中恢复过来。如果你继续治疗，你会感觉更好。"

Communicate the information that treatment is effective to the patient. For example, tell the patient, "Research shows that mental health treatment can help people recover from suicidal ideation or feelings. If you follow the treatment, you will feel better."

向患者解释出院后多久必须回医院复诊。

Explain when a return visit to the hospital is warranted.

为患者提供准确的当地危机干预中心或危机干预热线的信息，包括口头和书面信息。在离开医院之前,协助患者打电话给危机干预中心。

Provide verbal and written information identifying the local crisis center or crisis line. Assist the patient in making a call to the crisis center before leaving hospital.

使用教学反馈技巧确保患者及其家人理解所提供的信息。例如:"我们谈到了重要的后续随访计划。你能告诉我你回家后会做些什么吗?""我想确认一下我是否将这些信息都解释清楚了。你能用自己的话向我解释一遍吗?"

Use teach-back techniques to ensure the patient and his/her family understand the information provided. For example: "We talked about important things about next steps. Can you tell me what you'll do when you get home?" "I want to be sure I explained everything clearly. Can you please explain it back to me in your own words?"

同情和尊重患者自主权和隐私权。简要的患者教育干预的目标是给患者康复的希望并减少病耻感和羞耻感。

Show empathy and respect for patient autonomy and privacy. The goal of the Brief Patient Education intervention is to instill hope of recovery and to reduce stigma and shame.

提供书面教育材料,包括社区资源清单。

Provide written educational materials, including a list of community resources.

3.2.2 致命自杀方式的限制

3.2.2 Lethal Means Counseling

在致命性自杀方式的限制干预中,医护人员在评估有自杀风险的患者时应询问其是否可以获得农药或其他致命性自杀方式(例如处方药),并与患者及其朋友、家人或门诊医护人员一起讨论限制这些自杀方式的方法,直到患者不再有自杀倾向。

In the Lethal Means Counseling intervention, the provider assesses whether a patient with suicide risk has access to pesticide or other lethal means (e.g., prescription medications), and works with the patient and his/her friends, family, or outpatient provider to discuss ways to limit this access until the patient is no longer feeling suicidal.

尽管我们无法阻止患者包括自杀在内的所有自伤行为,但将患者安全作为重中之重,并贯穿评估和治疗的始终,有利于将患者的危险行为降至最低。

Although it is impossible to prevent all self-injurious actions including actual suicide, it is critically important to attend to the patient's safety and work to minimize self-endangering behavior throughout the evaluation and treatment process.

在临床实际中,在进行初步评估时可能需要采取一些干预措施来保障患者的安全。例如,在急诊科或者住院部,具体的干预措施可能包括一对一地对患者进行观察,或者通过监控持续观察,从患者房间移除可能的危险物品,以及保管患者的财物(因为钱包和背包内可能有武器、打火机或火柴、药物或其他可能的有毒物质)。

In actual practice, some interventions may be needed to address the patient's safety while the initial evaluation proceeds. For example, in emergency or inpatient settings, specific interventions may include ordering observation of the patient on a one-to-one basis or by continuous closed-circuit television monitoring, removing potentially hazardous items from the patient's room, and securing the patient's belongings (since purses and backpacks may contain weapons, cigarette lighters or matches, and medications or other potentially toxic substances).

如果患者需要封闭治疗,也建议进行连续观察。一些机构通过搜身或用金属探测器扫描患者来搜查可能的危险物品。在其他情况下,例如有躁动、不合作、中毒或伴有躯体疾病的患者,完成精神检查或者自杀评估后再处理可能会错过重要的治疗时间窗。在这种情况下,精神科医生需要利用现有的信息做出临床判断,并在此期间采取一切措施来保障患者的安全。

If restraints are indicated, continuous observation is also recommended. Some institutions screen patients for potentially dangerous items by searching patients or scanning them with metal detectors. In other circumstances, such as with agitated, uncooperative, intoxicated, or medically ill patients, significant time may elapse before it will be possible to complete a full psychiatric evaluation, including a suicide assessment. Under such conditions, the psychiatrist needs to use the information that is available to make a clinical judgment, with steps being taken to enhance the patient's safety in the interim.

实施步骤:

①告诉患者及其朋友或家人自杀风险有时会突然增加,因此在这些风险增加的时期考虑患者可获得的致命性自杀方式至关重要。

Action Steps:

① Tell the patient and his or her friends or family that suicide risk can sometimes escalate rapidly, so it is important to consider the patient's access to lethal means during these periods of increased risk.

②向患者及其支持者询问患者是否有机会获得致命性自杀方式,特别是农药。如果患者可以接触农药,请询问具体位置(例如,衣柜、汽车、阁楼)。

②Ask the patient and his or her supporters about the patient's access to lethal means, particularly pesticide. If the patient has access to pesticide, ask about the location (e.g., closet, car, attic).

③为可获得致命性自杀方式的患者提供适当的咨询。有关在简要咨询中需要涵盖的要点列表,请参考从"方式的重要性"(一项由哈佛大学公共卫生学院伤害控制中心发起的自杀预防项目)获得的医护人员版本的致命性自杀方式的咨询建议书。

③Provide appropriate counseling to the patients who may have access to lethal means. For a list of points that needs to be covered in brief counseling, see the paramedic version of the fatal suicide counseling recommendation available from The Importance of Means, a suicide prevention program sponsored by the Center for Injury Control at the Harvard School of Public Health.

④确定限制致命自杀方式的策略,例如在自杀危机结束前将农药等存放在朋友家中,并允许家庭成员将药物上锁保存并保管钥匙,在必要时由家属分配药物以防止患者过量服用。

④Identify strategies for limiting access to lethal means, such as storing pesticide at a friend's house until the suicidal crisis has passed, and allowing a family member to keep medications under lock and key and dispense them as necessary in order to prevent self-poisoning.

3.2.3 确定治疗环境

3.2.3 Determine a Treatment Setting

治疗环境包括一系列不同级别的医疗服务,从非自愿住院治疗到局部住院治疗和密集门诊治疗,再到普通门诊治疗。一般而言,患者应在限制性最小但最有可能保证安全性和有效性的环境中接受治疗。此外,在整个治疗过程中,应持续不断地重新评估最佳治疗环境和患者从不同水平的护理中获益的能力。

Treatment settings include a series of possible levels of care, from involuntary hospitalizations to partial hospital and intensive outpatient programs, more typical ambulatory settings. In general, patients should be treated in the setting that is least restrictive yet most likely to prove safe and effective. In addition, the optimal treatment setting and the patient's ability to benefit from a different level of care should be reevaluated on an ongoing basis throughout the course of treatment.

合适治疗环境的选择通常会在医护人员评估患者的临床情况后进行,包括特定的精神障碍和症状(例如,绝望、冲动、焦虑)、症状的严重程度、功能水平、可获得的支持系统以及如何给患者一个活下去的理由。

The choice of an appropriate site of treatment will generally occur after the medical staff evaluates the patient's clinical condition, including specific psychiatric disorders and symptoms(e.g., hopelessness, impulsiveness, anxiety), symptom severity, levels of functioning, available support systems, and activities that give the patient a reason to live.

医护人员还应该考虑当前的自杀倾向是否与人际关系危机有关,如最近的分离、失去亲人或其他创伤。显然,自杀风险的评估将是选择治疗环境的一个重要组成部分,并且还应考虑到自杀患者对他人的危险性。

The medical staff should also consider whether or not the current suicidality is related to an interpersonal crisis such as a recent separation, loss of a loved one, or other trauma. The estimate of suicide risk will obviously be an important component of the choice of treatment setting, and the potential for dangerousness to others should also be taken into consideration.

在某些临床情况下,是否住院治疗主要取决于患者对自身或其他人的潜在危险程度,即使无法获得更多的病史或者如果患者不能配合精神检查(例如,在极度激惹、精神病性症状或紧张症)。同时,必须权衡住院等强化干预措施的益处及其可能产生的不利影响(如就业中断、经济和其他社会心理压力、持续的社会耻辱感等)。

Under some clinical circumstances, a decision for hospitalization may need to be made on the basis of high potential dangerousness to self or others, even if additional history is unavailable or if the patient is unable to cooperate with the psychiatric evaluation (e.g., in the presence of extreme agitation, psychosis, or catatonia). At the same time, the benefits of intensive interventions such as hospitalization must be weighed against their possible negative effects (e.g., disruption of employment, financial and other psychosocial stress, persistent societal stigma).

决定是否让患者进入治疗环境的其他方面因素还包括患者的自理能力、是否能理解各种治疗的风险和益处、了解在危机中应该做些什么(例如,联系家庭成员或其他支持人员、精神科医生,以寻求急诊医疗)、能否向精神科医生提供可靠的反馈,以及是否能配合治疗方案的制定和实施。因此,选择一个特定的治疗环境将不完全取决于自杀风险的估计,而是取决于能否在多种影响因素间找到平衡。

Other aspects to be incorporated into the determination of a treatment setting include the patient's ability to provide adequate self-care, understand the risks and benefits of various treatment approaches, understand what to do in a crisis (e.g., contacting family members or other support persons, and the psychiatrist, seeking emergency care), give reliable feedback to the psychiatrist, and cooperate with treatment planning and implementation. Consequently, choice of a specific treatment setting will not depend entirely on the estimate of suicide risk but rather on the balance between these various elements.

住院时间长短同样应该由患者在相对宽松的治疗环境中安全地接受所需治疗的能力决定。此外,在患者过渡到限制性较低的治疗环境之前,患者自杀风险和精神症状的评估均应有所改善,并趋于稳定。

The hospital length of stay should similarly be determined by the ability of the patient to receive the needed care safely in a less intensive environment. In addition, before the patient is transitioned to a less restrictive setting, the patient's condition should show evidence of being improved and more stable both in the estimated level of suicide risk and in the symptoms of any associated psychiatric disorders.

如果自杀意念和自杀企图长期反复出现,并且患者自己能意识到这一点,那么较弱强度的治疗可能更适合这类自杀患者。对于这样的患者,自杀意念可能是对"失落"的特征性反应或者是患者对心理应激的一种应对方式。

Less intensive treatment may be more appropriate if suicidal ideation or attempts are part of a chronic, repetitive cycle and the patient is aware of the chronicity. For such patients, suicidal ideation may be a characteristic response to disappointment or a way to cope with psychological distress.

如果患者病史中只有自杀意念但没有自杀意图,并且目前正在接受治疗,那么即使有严重的精神症状,在医院外继续治疗的益处也可能大于住院治疗可能造成的不利影响。

If the patient has a history of suicidal ideation without suicidal intent and an ongoing doctor-patient relationship, the benefits of continued treatment outside the hospital may outweigh the possible detrimental effects of hospitalization even in the presence of serious psychiatric symptoms.

当考虑住院时,自杀的风险并不是唯一的考虑因素。患者在医院可能会感到羞辱或害怕,而不是感受到情绪的缓解。住院还可能与现实生活中的应激因素有关,应激因素包括接受住院治疗的社会和经济负担。

When considering hospitalization, suicide risk is not the only factor to take into account. Patients may feel humiliated or frightened in the hospital rather than experience a sense of emotional relief. Hospitalization can also be associated with realistic life stressors, including the social and financial burdens of having received inpatient treatment.

对于一些患者,在诸如住院病房这样的限制性环境中进行治疗可能会使患者产生并加重功能退化,进而加重自杀意念,形成恶性循环,导致需要更多的限制性治疗。人格障碍的患者这种情况尤为突出,如果他们没有得到支持来承受痛苦的感受,就会遭受慢性疾病的折磨。

For some patients, treatment in a restrictive setting such as an inpatient unit may foster dependency and a regressive, vicious cycle of intensifying suicidal ideation. They require ever more restrictive care. Such individuals, most notably those with personality disorders, suffer chronic morbidity if they are never supportively challenged to bear painful feelings.

此外,一些患者可能会因住院获得正性自我强化,为了再次住院会反复伤害自己。精神科住院治疗也可能给患者、家庭成员、治疗师和医护人员不切实际的期望。通常,住院的请求源于家属或相关人员对患者当时情况的不满。

In addition, some patients may gain positive reinforcement from hospitalization and repeatedly harm themselves with the goal of regaining admission. Psychiatric hospitalization may also arouse unrealistic expectations in patients, family members, therapists, and medical staff members. Often, a plea for hospitalization comes from a sense of exasperation on the part of an individual involved with the patient's situation.

当住院治疗不能满足这些不切实际的期望时,相关的幻想破灭可能会导致绝望,并对未来的治疗关系产生负面影响。住院过程本身也可能导致患者不信任精神卫生专业人员,特别是在非自愿住院的情况下。

When hospital treatment does not meet these unrealistic expectations, the associated disillusionment may contribute to hopelessness and have a negative effect on future therapeutic relationships. The inpatient admission process itself may also cause the patient to mistrust mental health professionals, particularly when hospitalization occurs on an involuntary basis.

因此,临床医生的关键责任是在入院前和住院期间权衡住院的风险和益处(特别是关于治疗性通行证与特权级别的决定),并最后慎重考虑出院时间。此外,关于个人隐私和自主权(包括在最低限制的环境中接受治疗的权利),必须以权衡自伤或他伤的潜在风险作为前提。

Thus, the clinician's key responsibility is to weigh the risks and benefits of hospitalization before and during admission (especially around decisions related to therapeutic passes and privilege levels) and ultimately carefully consider the discharge time. Moreover, a person's right to privacy and self-determination (which includes the right to be treated in the least restrictive environment) must be balanced against the issue of potential dangerousness to self or others.

3.2.4 制定治疗计划

3.2.4 Develop a Plan of Treatment

有自杀意念、计划或行为的患者可能受益于多种治疗。如果患者有自杀风险,那么整合一系列生物和心理社会疗法的治疗计划可能会增加治疗的成功率。选择治疗方案时须权衡各种治疗的利弊,并了解患者的偏好。

Patients with suicidal ideation, plans, or behaviors may benefit from a variety of treatments. If the patient is at risk for suicide, a plan that integrates a range of biological and psychosocial therapies may increase the likelihood of a successful outcome. Treatment options should be chosen by weighing the pros and cons of various treatments and knowing the patient's preferences.

此外,治疗决定应该随着新信息的出现和患者临床状态的改变而不断重新评估。对于正在接受治疗的患者,如果患者的自杀想法或自杀行为出现或减少,即需要调整现有的治疗计划。

In addition, treatment decisions should be continually reassessed as new information becomes available, and the patient's clinical status changes. For patients in ongoing treatment, this may mean that existing treatment plans will require modification as suicidal ideas or behaviors emerge or wane.

因此,制定治疗计划是一个反复的过程,在这个过程中精神科医生与患者合作,并根据患者的反应和偏好来实施和修改治疗。根据临床情况,治疗计划过程可能涉及家庭成员或其他重要支持(例如,社区居民或社工、病例管理人员等)。

Thus, treatment planning is an iterative process in which the psychiatrist works with the patient to implement and modify treatments over time, depending on the patient's responses and preferences. Depending on the clinical circumstances, it may be important for the treatment planning process to include his family members or other significant support (e.g., community residence or adult home providers, case management staff).

应该提醒医护人员的是,在制定治疗计划时不要以"消除"自杀风险为目标,这是不可能做到的。相反,治疗的目标应该包括以减少自杀风险为主要目标的综合治疗方法。由于有自杀行为的人通常有轴Ⅰ和轴Ⅱ精神障碍,降低风险通常涉及治疗相关的精神障碍。

Medical staff should be cautioned against developing a treatment plan in which the stated goal is to "eliminate" suicide risk; this is impossible to do. Instead, the goals of treatment should include a comprehensive approach to treatment with the major focus directed at reducing risk. Since individuals with suicidal behaviors often have axis I and axis II disorders, reducing risk frequently involves treating an associated psychiatric illness.

鉴于有自杀行为的患者常伴有酒精和毒品滥用,在治疗计划中解决物质滥用的问题尤为重要。在为自杀患者制定治疗计划时,还需要考虑躯体疾病及其治疗方法。

Given the high rates of comorbid alcohol and substance use among patients with suicidal behaviors, it is particularly important to address substance use disorders in the treatment plan. Medical disorders and treatments for those disorders will also need to be considered in developing a plan of treatment for the patient with suicidal behaviors.

在治疗的早期阶段,可能需要更密切的随访以便为患者提供支持,并监测和迅速开始相关症状的治疗,如焦虑、失眠或绝望。此外,在疾病的早期阶段,否认症状和缺乏对治疗的相关认识可能是最突出的问题,因此,需要针对这些问题进行具体的患者教育和支持性心理治疗。

In the early stages of treatment, more intense follow-up may be needed to provide support for the patient as well as to monitor and rapidly institute treatment for relevant symptoms such as anxiety, insomnia, or hopelessness. In addition, during the early stages of illness, denial of symptoms and lack of insight into the need for treatment are likely to be most prominent, therefore, specific education and supportive psychotherapy are required to target these issues.

了解患者过去对心理应激的反应、是否有使用致命性自杀方式的倾向、可用的外部资源、死亡幻想和现实检验能力,可能有助于临床医生权衡患者的优势和弱点,也有助于制定更优的治疗计划。

Appreciating the patient's past responses to stress, vulnerability to life-threatening affects, available external resources, death fantasies, and capacity for reality testing may help the clinician to weigh the strengths and vulnerabilities of the individual patient and may aid in the planning of treatment.

对于在门诊环境中接受治疗的患者,精神科医生也有必要参考患者指南,以预防患者出现自杀倾向加重和就诊期间其他与自杀相关的症状加重而导致自杀风险增加。

For patients treated in ambulatory settings, it is also important for the psychiatrist to review the patient guidelines for managing exacerbations of suicidal tendencies or other symptoms that may occur between scheduled sessions and could contribute to increased suicide risk.

3.2.5 安全计划

3.2.5 Safety Planning

安全计划干预,即医护人员与患者合作制定患者在自杀危机之前或期间可以使用的应对策略和可获得资源列表。该计划要求简短,用患者自己的话表述,易于阅读。大多数安全计划中涉及的主题包括以下内容:

- 患者个人警示信号;
- 内部应对策略;
- 能帮助患者脱离危机的方法;
- 能够提供支持的家庭成员或朋友;
- 可以寻求帮助的专业人士和机构;
- 保障环境安全的方法。

In the Safety Planning Intervention, the medical staff work with a patient to develop a list of coping strategies and resources that he or she can use before or during suicidal crises. The plan is brief, in the patient's own words, and easy to read. Topics addressed in most safety plans include:

- The patient's individual warning signs;
- Internal coping strategies;
- Ways to distract oneself from the crisis;
- Family members or friends who can provide support;
- Professionals and agencies to contact for help;
- Ways to make the environment safe.

安全计划可以在纸上或使用移动应用程序完成——如果患者有移动设备并且乐于使用。安全计划干预由 Barbara Stanley 博士和 Gregory K. Brown 博士开发。要点:安全计划不应与"安全合同"或"不自杀合同"混淆。没有证据表明这些合同是有效的,而且它们会提供虚假的安全感。

Safety plans may be done on paper or use a mobile phone app—if the patient has a mobile device and is comfortable to use it for this purpose. The Safety Planning Intervention was developed by Barbara Stanley, PhD, and Gregory K. Brown, PhD. Important: Safety planning should not be confused with contracts for safety or no-suicide contracts. There is no evidence that these contracts are effective, and they can provide a false sense of security.

实施步骤：

①回顾《降低自杀风险的安全计划治疗手册》：该手册为退伍军人版本，可以将此作为制定"安全计划干预"的蓝本。本手册中的指南适用于所有患者群体。

②告诉患者我们建议制定安全计划。请与患者共同决定：是否由我们和患者共同制定该计划，或者患者独立制定计划，然后在出院前与我们共同审阅。在患者允许的情况下，让他/她的家人、朋友和/或同伴参与进来。

③使用"安全计划资源"中列出的工具之一来制定安全计划。

④确定使用安全计划的潜在障碍或困难，并确定如何克服这些障碍。

⑤告诉患者，虽然安全计划对于应对治疗环境之外的自杀想法或自杀感受很重要，但是接受门诊心理诊疗可以明确使他/她产生自杀倾向的问题。

⑥指导患者与门诊医护人员一起审查安全计划。为医护及患者均提供一份副本。

Action Steps：

①Review the Safety Plan Treatment Manual to Reduce Suicide Risk：Veteran Version for an orientation to this intervention. The guidance in this manual is suitable for all patient populations.

②Tell the patient that we recommend developing a safety plan. Decide together if the patient needs our help to develop it or if he or she will develop the plan independently and then review it with us before discharge. With the patient's permission，involve his or her family，friends，and/or a peer specialist.

③Use one of the tools listed under Safety Planning Resources to develop a safety plan.

④Identify potential barriers or obstacles of using the safety plan and determine how to overcome them.

⑤Tell the patient that although safety plans are important for coping with suicidal ideation or feelings outside of the treatment setting，getting outpatient mental health care can address what's making him or her feel suicidal.

⑥Instruct the patient to review the safety plan with an outpatient provider. Provide a copy for each.

最初，"自杀预防合同"有时也被称为"无伤害合同"，旨在加强患者自杀风险的管理。虽然在管理式的医疗时代，自杀预防合同越来越多地被用于有自杀风险的患者，但患者是否愿意签订"自杀预防合同"不能作为患者出院/入院的绝对指标。

At first，the suicide prevention contract，which is sometimes known as a no-harm contract，was intended to facilitate management of the patient at suicide risk.

Although in the era of managed care, suicide prevention contracts are increasingly being used with patients with suicide risk, the patient's willingness (or reluctance) to enter into a suicide prevention contract should not be viewed as an absolute indicator of suitability for discharge or hospitalization.

此外,由于自杀预防合同的效用是基于主观信念而非客观证据,它被高估为临床或风险管理技术。此外,自杀预防合同不是法律文件,在法律诉讼中不能用作无罪证据。因此,自杀预防合同不能也不应该取代全面的自杀风险评估。

In addition, since the utility of the suicide prevention contract is based on subjective belief rather than objective evidence, it is overvalued as a clinical or risk management technique. Furthermore, the suicide prevention contract is not a legal document and cannot be used as exculpatory evidence in the event of litigation. Thus, the suicide prevention contract cannot and should not take the place of a thorough suicide risk assessment.

虽然自杀预防合同常用于临床实践,但没有研究表明它能有效减少自杀。事实上,对自杀未遂和自杀死亡的住院患者的研究表明,相当多的人在自杀行为发生时都曾签订自杀预防合同。

Although suicide prevention contracts are commonly used in clinical practice, no studies have shown their effectiveness in reducing suicide. In fact, studies of suicide attempters and of inpatients who died by suicide have shown that a significant number had a suicide prevention contract in place at the time of their suicidal act.

因此,尽管口头和书面的自杀预防合同已被推荐作为评估治疗关系的辅助手段,但也应该清楚它们的局限性。同时,过度依赖患者的自杀预防合同可能会错误地降低临床警惕性,自杀合同并不能改变患者的自杀状态。

Consequently, although verbal and written suicide prevention contracts have each been proposed as aids to assessing the therapeutic alliance, their limitations should also be clearly understood. At the same time, undue reliance on a patient's suicide prevention contract may falsely lower clinical vigilance without altering the patient's suicidal state.

一些临床医生通过患者是否愿意正式建立医患联盟的口头或书面合同来考量患者的自杀意图。例如,在讨论自杀预防合同时,一些患者会公开表明,如果出现自我毁灭的冲动时,他们无法确定他们能否(或想要)打电话给精神科医生或其他治疗团队成员。

Some clinicians gauge the patient's suicidal intent by his or her willingness to formalize the alliance with a written or an oral contract. For example, when discussing a suicide prevention contract, some patients will state openly that they cannot be sure that they can (or will want to) call the psychiatrist or other treatment team members if self-destructive impulses threaten.

拒绝自杀预防合同的患者表明他们认为治疗关系不是最理想的或者他们感觉无法遵守此类合同。因此,拒绝签署自杀合同的患者提醒临床医生应该重新评估治疗关系和自杀风险水平。

Patients who reject a suicide prevention contract are communicating that they see the therapeutic alliance as suboptimal or that they feel unable to adhere to such a contract. Consequently, patients who refuse to commit to contracts against suicide put the clinician on notice that the therapeutic alliance and the level of suicide risk should be reassessed.

另一种自杀合同是米勒等人提出的基于知情同意的原则,通过与患者进行有关治疗和管理方案的风险和益处的讨论,来评估患者建立和维持治疗关系的能力。在住院患者中,这种讨论可以提高医护人员在患者心目中的存在感,并教育患者在应对自杀冲动时可以选择向他们求助。

An alternative approach to suicide prevention contracts proposed by Miller *et al.* relies on the basic tenets of informed consent and discusses the risks and benefits of treatment and management options with the patient as a means of assessing his or her ability to develop and maintain a therapeutic alliance. In inpatient setting, such discussions can emphasize the availability of the clinical staff and be used as a way to educate the patient about options for dealing with suicidal impulses.

无论潜在的优势如何,自杀预防合同只有在治疗关系稳固时生效。因此,对于新的患者,精神科医生可能没有足够的时间进行充分的评估或评估患者建立治疗关系的能力,依靠自杀预防合同来预防自杀是没有现实基础的。

Regardless of their potential advantages, suicide prevention contracts are only as reliable as the state of the therapeutic alliance. Thus, with a new patient, the psychiatrist may not have sufficient time to make an adequate assessment or to evaluate the patient's capacity to form a therapeutic alliance. There is no practical basis to rely on suicide prevention contracts to prevent suicide.

因此,不建议在急诊或者与新入院和不了解病情的住院患者签订自杀预防合同。此外,由于疾病的严重程度不同,处于危机中的患者可能无法遵守合同。对于躁动、有精神病性障碍或冲动的患者或当患者受到精神活性物质影响时,使用自杀预防合同也是不明智的。对于这类患者,当出现自杀行为时,医护人员必须时刻注意持续进行自杀评估的必要性。

As a result, the use of suicide prevention contracts in emergency settings or with newly admitted and unknown inpatients is not recommended. Furthermore, patients in crisis may not be able to adhere to a contract because of the severity of their illness. It is also unwise to use suicide prevention contracts for patients who are restless, have psychotic disorders or impulsivity, or when patients are under the influence of psychoactive substances. For these patients, as for all patients presenting with suicidal behaviors, the medical staff must be ever mindful of the need for ongoing suicide assessments.

3.2.6 患者安全和自杀风险的再评估
3.2.6 Reassess Safety and Suicide Risk

自杀意念的起伏变化是自杀预防的难点之一,这就要求医护人员持续反复评估自杀。虽然不需要在每次访谈中对患者进行完整的自杀评估,但医护人员应该通过合理的判断来明确患者当前自杀风险所需的重复自杀评估范围。

The waxing and waning nature of suicidality is one of the difficult challenges in the care of the suicidal patient and often requires that suicide assessments be repeated over time. Although a full suicide assessment is not required at each encounter with patient, the medical staff should use reasonable judgment in determining the extent of the repeat assessment needed to estimate the patient's current suicide risk.

在住院患者中,在治疗的关键阶段(例如,护理级别的变化、精神状态突然改变、出院前)应该进行反复多次评估。当多次评估完成后,医务人员经常会发现,最初报告具有致命意图的自杀意念患者在随后访问中不再报告自杀意念。

In inpatient settings, repeat suicide assessments should occur at critical stages of treatment (e.g., with a change in level of privilege, abrupt change in mental state, and before discharge). When a reassessment is done, the medical staff often find that the patient who initially reported suicidal ideation with lethal intent no longer reports suicidal ideation at a subsequent visit.

如前所述,要准确预测哪些患者的自杀意念是否会再次出现是不可能的,也很难预测哪些患者会否认自己存在自杀意念。尽管如此,如果发现患者较高的自杀风险,则必须通过评估计划来明确风险并记录。该计划可能包括治疗环境的变化(如护理级别或观察水平的变化)、治疗方案的变化(药物治疗或心理治疗的变化)或兼有以上两种变化。

As stated earlier, it is not possible to predict which individuals with recent suicidal ideation will experience it again, nor which patients will deny suicidal ideation even when it is present. Nonetheless, if a patient is assessed as being at a high risk for suicide, a plan to address this risk must be implemented and documented. This plan may include changes in the setting of care or levels of observation, changes in medication therapy or psychotherapy, or both kinds of changes.

尤其是近期有严重自杀意念的患者应特别谨慎对待。对于抑郁障碍患者的自杀意念,监测其他抑郁症状可能有助于评估自杀风险。

Patients with a recent onset of severe suicidal ideation should be treated with particular caution. For those experiencing suicidal ideation in the context of an underlying depressive disorder, it can be useful to monitor other depressive symptoms.

医护人员还需要注意可能与自杀风险增加相关的其他症状,如绝望、焦虑、失眠或命令性幻觉;可能与风险急剧增加相关的行为包括放弃财产、准备法律或财务事宜(如确定遗嘱、签订授权委托书等)、传递自杀意图或具有"告别"意义的信息。

The medical staff also needs to be mindful of other symptoms that may be associated with increased suicide risk, such as hopelessness, anxiety, insomnia, or command hallucinations. Behaviors that may be associated with an acute increase in risk include giving away possessions, readying legal or financial affairs (e.g., finalizing a will, assigning a power of attorney), or communicating suicidal intentions or "goodbye" messages.

对于当前治疗有效,或者处于维持治疗康复期的患者,当出现病情变化,包括症状的复燃或复发,或是出现重大的不良生活事件时,应该对患者进行自杀风险评估。在这种情况下,应通过改变治疗计划以应对新出现的自杀风险。

Patients who are responding to ongoing treatment or who are in remission with continuation or maintenance treatment should be assessed for suicide risk when there is evidence of an abrupt clinical change, a relapse or recurrence, or some major adverse life event. In this context, the new emergence of suicidality should be responded to by an alteration of the treatment plan.

治疗计划如何调整应视临床情况而定,可包括治疗环境或观察水平的调整、增加随访次数、调整药物治疗或心理治疗、将患者重要的联系人纳入治疗计划,以及进行相关咨询等。当临床状态的变化或获得新的患者信息时,医护人员还必须准备重新评估患者的精神障碍诊断,并评估治疗关系的性质和牢固程度。

The nature of this alteration depends on the clinical situation and can include a change in treatment setting or levels of observation, increased visits, a change of medication or psychotherapeutic approaches, inclusion of a significant other person, and consultation. With changes in clinical status or as new information becomes available, the medical staff must also be prepared to reevaluate the patient's psychiatric diagnosis and also evaluate the nature and strength of the therapeutic alliance.

（1）出现自杀危机的患者。

（1）Patients in a Suicidal Crisis.

有时正在进行治疗的患者突然出现自杀危机,医护人员必须立即做出反应。可能需要直接与患者家人或其他重要联系人进行沟通。在紧急情况下,可能有必要通过电话追踪或让警察介入。

Sometimes patients undergoing treatment suddenly have a suicide crisis and the medical staff have to respond immediately. There may be communications directly with the patient' family, or significant others. In urgent situations, it may be necessary to have telephone calls traced or involve the police.

医护人员面临的挑战不仅是评估自杀危机的严重程度,还要评估与患者联系的信息内容和信息来源。为了更好地评估病情,如果可能的话,直接与患者沟通至关重要。此外,医护人员应该始终注意与保密协议有关的问题,并且只有在为了确保患者安全的特殊情况下才能违反保密协议。

The challenge for the medical staff is not only to evaluate the extent of the emergency but also to assess the content of the communication and its source. To better assess the situation, it is critical to communicate with the patient directly, if at all possible. In addition, the medical staff should remain mindful of issues relating to confidentiality and breach confidentiality only to the extent needed to address the patient's safety.

在某些情况下,医务人员可能需要将自杀患者转诊到急诊科进行评估或住院治疗。此时,医务人员与急诊科的精神障碍评估员进行沟通非常重要。尽管由于情况紧急,这种沟通并不总是可能的,但这种沟通能告知医院工作人员该患者情况的紧急性。

Under some circumstances, the medical staff may need to refer a suicidal patient to an emergency department for evaluation or hospitalization. When doing so, it is important for the medical staff to communicate with the psychiatric evaluator in the emergency department. Although such communication may not always be possible because of the exigencies of the emergency situation, such contact does provide hospital personnel with the context for the emergency.

特别是当患者是被警察带到医院时,到达急诊后,部分患者会否认转诊的症状和原因。充分提供有关急诊科转诊原因以及患者既往和现病史信息有助于急诊科评估人员为患者提供安全且合适的治疗环境。

Particularly when a patient is brought to the hospital by police, it is not unusual for the patient to minimize the symptoms and reasons for the referral after arriving in the emergency setting. Adequate information about the reasons for the emergency department referral and about the patient's previous and recent history can be crucial in helping the emergency department evaluator determine a safe and appropriate setting for treatment.

当转诊精神科医生建议患者住院治疗时,建议住院的原因也应该告知急诊科评估员,由这些评估员最终确定患者是否需要住院。

When hospitalization is recommended by the referring psychiatrist, the reasons for that recommendation should similarly be communicated to the emergency department evaluator who will be making the final determination about the need for hospital admission.

(2)慢性自杀患者。

(2)Patients with Chronic Suicidality.

部分患者的自伤行为和/或自杀会长期反复出现,导致医疗保健系统需要经常与其联系以反复评估自杀风险。需要认识到自伤行为可能与自杀意图有关,也可能无关。

For some individuals, self-injurious behaviors and/or suicidality are chronic and repetitive, resulting in frequent contacts with the health care system for assessment of suicide potential. It is important to recognize that self-injurious behaviors may or may not be associated with suicidal intent.

尽管自伤行为有时被描述为旨在达到其他目的的"姿态"(例如,通过住院治疗获得关注或逃避责任等),患者对此类行为的动机却大不相同。例如,患者并非想结束自己生命,只是通过故意伤害自己表达愤怒、缓解焦虑或紧张、产生"正常或自我控制"的感觉、终止人格解体的状态、分散注意力或惩罚自己。

Although self-injurious behaviors are sometimes characterized as "gestures" aimed at achieving secondary gains (e.g., receiving attention, avoiding responsibility through hospitalization), patients' motivations for such behaviors are quite different. For example, without having any desire for death, individuals may intentionally injure themselves to express anger, relieve anxiety or tension, generate a feeling of "normality or self-control," terminate a state of depersonalization, or distract or punish themselves.

将此类"姿态"行为一概而论也是有偏颇的,因为当与轻微的自我伤害相关联时,自杀企图可能被淡化。即使在患者没有自杀意图的情况下,自我毁灭性行为也可能导致患者意外死亡。此外,过去或现在仅有非致命性自伤行为并不排除患者没有严重甚至致命的自杀意念、自杀计划或自杀企图。

Conceptualizing such behaviors as "gestures" is also problematic because suicide attempts may be downplayed when associated with minimal self-harm. Self-destructive acting out can also result in accidentally lethal self-destructive behaviors even in the absence of suicidal intent. Furthermore, a past or current history of non-lethal self-injurious behaviors does not preclude development of suicidal ideas, plans, or attempts with serious intent and lethality.

事实上,在有自杀意图的自杀未遂者中,那些既往出现无自杀意图的自伤行为的患者,其自杀企图的客观致命性更有可能被低估,并更有可能伴随高自杀风险的相关症状。

In fact, among suicide attempters with suicidal intent, those who also had histories of self-injurious behaviors without suicidal intent were more likely to underestimate the objective lethality of their attempt and to have symptoms associated with greater suicide risk.

因此,在评估慢性自伤行为时,重要的是确定自伤行为是否伴有自杀意图,如果二者相互关联,则须明确其发生的频率和程度。此外,没有自杀意图或轻微的自伤行为不应作为医护人员忽视其他可能增加自杀风险证据的理由。

Thus, in assessing chronic self-injurious behaviors, it is important to determine whether suicidal intent is present with self-injury and, if so, to what extent and with what frequency. In addition, an absence of suicidal intent or a minimal degree of self-injury should not lead the medical staff to overlook other evidence of increased suicide risk.

对于有慢性自伤行为倾向的患者,每种行为都需要根据当前情况进行评估;对于自伤行为没有特定的治疗方式推荐。例如,有时门诊管理最合适,而某些情况可能需要住院治疗。

For patients who are prone to chronic self-injurious behavior, each act needs to be assessed in the context of the current situation; there is not a single response to self-injurious behaviors that can be recommended. For example, there are times when outpatient management is most appropriate; under other circumstances, hospitalization may be indicated.

一般来说,对于这类人群,住院治疗应该用于急性期控制,因为长期住院治疗可能会加剧依赖、功能退化和毁灭性行为。当伴有慢性自伤行为时,诸如辩证行为疗法之类的行为矫正技术可能会有所帮助。此外,在将患者转诊到另一个临床医生的时候,患者自杀风险可能会增加。

In general, for such individuals, hospitalization should be used for short-term stabilization, since prolonged hospital stays may potentiate dependency, regression, and acting-out behaviors. When chronic self-injurious behaviors are present, behavioral techniques such as dialectical behavior therapy can be helpful. In addition, at times when care of the patient is being transitioned to another clinician, the risk of suicidal behaviors may increase.

从诊断上讲,在表现出慢性自伤行为而没有相关自杀意图的患者中绝大多数可能有严重的人格障碍,特别是边缘型和反社会型人格障碍,这些个体也可能有共病惊恐障碍和创伤后应激障碍。患有分裂性情感障碍、双向情感障碍和精神分裂症的患者也可能出现这种情况,但这三种精神障碍的患者更常见的是伴有自杀意图的自杀想法或自杀企图。

Diagnostically, severe personality disorders, particularly borderline and antisocial personality disorders, predominate among patients who exhibit chronic self-injurious behaviors without associated suicidal intent. Such individuals may also have higher rates of comorbid panic disorder and post-traumatic stress disorder. Patients with schizo-affective disorder, bipolar disorder, and schizophrenia may also be represented, but more often such patients have ongoing thoughts of suicide or repeated suicide attempts in the presence of suicidal intent.

有证据表明共病人格障碍或物质使用障碍不仅会增加患者的自杀风险,还会降低疗效。例如,患有情感障碍和人格障碍的患者容易发生频繁的自杀危机、情绪不稳定和冲动控制障碍以及治疗依从性问题。因此,对于依从性差导致长期自杀风险的患者,医护人员应熟悉非自愿门诊治疗的法规。

There is evidence that the presence of comorbid personality disorders or substance use disorders not only increases suicide risk in these individuals, but also decreases treatment response. For example, patients with a combination of affective disorder and personality disorder are prone to frequent suicidal crises, difficulties with mood instability and impulse control, and problems with treatment adherence. Consequently, for patients whose nonadherence contributes to a chronic risk for suicide, medical staff should be familiar with statutes on involuntary outpatient treatment.

3.2.7 患者家属的相关教育

3.2.7 Education of the Patient's Family

作为治疗的一部分,大多数病人都能从症状和障碍的治疗以及所采用的治疗方法的健康教育中受益。在适当的情况下,如果患者允许,还应向相关家庭成员提供健康教育。

Most patients can benefit from education about the symptoms and disorders being treated as well as about the therapeutic approaches employed as part of the treatment plan. When appropriate, and with the patient's permission, education should also be provided to involved family members.

患者和家庭成员还可以从了解心理社会应激对自杀的影响,和其他诱发或加剧自杀和精神症状的因素中获益。关于现有治疗方案的健康教育可帮助患者或家属接受治疗、了解可能出现的药物副作用并坚持治疗。

Patients and family members can also benefit from an understanding of the role of psychosocial stressors and other disruptions in precipitating or exacerbating suicidality or symptoms of psychiatric disorders. Education regarding available treatment options will help patients or their families make informed decisions, anticipate side effects, and adhere to treatments.

还应该让患者或家属明白治疗的疗效可能会波动,预后也会因人而异。某些患者或家庭成员在治疗开始后可能因症状反复或症状暂时恶化而变得不知所措或精神崩溃。由于自杀患者往往对自己过于挑剔,症状的复发或恶化可能被视为个人失败的证据,应该让他们认识到,这是恢复过程的一部分。

Patients or their familyies also need to be advised that improvement is not linear and that recovery may be uneven. Certain patients or their family members may become overwhelmed or devastated by a recurrence of symptoms or a temporary worsening of symptoms after the initiation of treatment. Since suicidal patients tend to be overly critical of themselves, a recurrence or worsening of symptoms may be seen as evidence of personal failure; they need to be reassured that this can be part of the recovery process.

与患者直接讨论自杀现象也是有益的。当有自杀的家族史时,一些患者会觉得自杀是他们的命运。家庭成员死亡的年龄或家庭成员死亡的某个周年纪念日可能对部分患者具有特殊意义。

It is also useful to have an open discussion with the patient about the phenomenon of suicide. When there has been a family history of suicide, some patients will feel that it is their fate to die from suicide as well. The age at which a family member died or the specific anniversary of the family member's death may take on special significance for some patients.

对患者和家庭的教育应该强调,有自杀家族史的人可能会增加自杀的风险,但这并不意味着自杀是不可避免的。可以帮助教育患者和有关家庭成员如何识别症状,如失眠、绝望、焦虑或抑郁,这些症状可能预示着患者的临床状况在恶化。

Education for the patient and the family should emphasize that a family history of suicide may increase risk of suicide, but it does not make suicide inevitable. It can be helpful to educate the patient and involved family members about how to identify symptoms, such as insomnia, hopelessness, anxiety, or depression, that may herald a worsening of the patient's clinical condition.

此外,应鼓励患者和家属考虑过去曾与自杀有关的其他特定症状。而且,患者和家属应该意识到,自杀的意念可能会反复出现,如果出现自杀意念,他们应该尽快通知精神科医生或其他重要人员。

In addition, patients and their family members should be encouraged to think about other symptoms, specific to the individual patient, that have been associated with suicidality in the past. Furthermore, patients and their family members should be aware that suicidal ideation may return and that they should inform the psychiatrist or a significant other as soon as possible if that occurs.

同时还应公开讨论发生紧急情况时如何处理以及如何获得紧急救助。在某些情况下,这种讨论可能还包括解释让警察参与协助进行非自愿评估的方法。

There should also be an open discussion about what to do in the event of an emergency and how to obtain emergency services. Under some circumstances, this discussion may include an explanation of methods for involving the police to facilitate an involuntary evaluation.

部分家庭成员,尤其是边缘型人格障碍患者的家人,错误地将自杀企图或自杀意图的沟通视为患者"操纵性"或"寻求关注"的行为。因此,向家庭成员提供有关此类患者终生自杀风险的教育,并帮助家庭成员学习如何在患者经历自杀危机时以一种有益和积极的方式应对是很重要的。

Some family members, particularly those of patients with borderline personality disorder, mistakenly view suicide attempts or communications of suicidal intent as "manipulative" or "attention-seeking" behaviors. Thus, it is important to provide family members with education about the lifetime risks of suicide in such patients and to help their family members learn ways to respond in a helpful and positive manner when the patient is experiencing a suicidal crisis.

此外,还应关注自杀患者家属的心理状态。自杀者家属更容易发生生理和心理障碍,并且他们自身的自杀风险高于普通人群。虽然对自杀者家属的系统研究相对较少,但现有研究表明在亲人自杀后,自杀者家属的情绪、社会和身体状况会显著变化。

In addition, attention should also be paid to the psychological status of the relatives of suicide patients. The survivors of suicide are more vulnerable to physical and psychological disorders and are at an increased risk of suiciding themselves. Although there are relatively few systematic studies of adult bereavement after suicide, existing studies suggest that emotional, social, and physical conditions of survivors are significantly changed after the suicide of a relative.

在自杀后的6个月内,45%的自杀者家属精神状况恶化,其中20%的躯体状况变差。在此期间,抑郁症、创伤后应激、内疚感和羞耻感以及躯体症状普遍存在,在已故儿童的父母中更为严重。

Within 6 months after a suicide, 45% of bereaved adults report mental deterioration, with physical deterioration in 20%. Symptoms of depression, post-traumatic stress, guilt, and shame as well as somatic complaints are prevalent during that period and are more severe among the parents of deceased children.

虽然大多数幸存者承认在亲人自杀后6个月内最需要干预,但只有25%的人寻求精神心理治疗。尽管就诊率很低,但从长远来看,大多数幸存者远期适应良好。

While the majority of bereaved adults within 6 months after a suicide acknowledge a need for intervention, only approximately 25% seek psychiatric treatment. Despite this low rate of treatment, the majority of bereaved adults adapt well in the long term.

关于年轻自杀幸存者的数据是最全面的。这些数据表明,在朋友或兄弟姐妹自杀后的6个月内,在失去亲人的年轻人中普遍存在重度抑郁和创伤后应激障碍症状。

The most comprehensive data on bereavement after suicide exist for youths. These data indicate that within 6 months after the suicide of a friend or sibling, symptoms of major depressive and post-traumatic stress disorders are prevalent among bereaved youths.

青少年在亲人自杀死亡后的远期预后(18个月)研究表明,在亲人自杀前患有抑郁症的青少年当中,重度抑郁症的发生率更高,在自杀后立即患抑郁症的青少年抑郁症发生率居中，在自杀后未立即患抑郁症的青少年抑郁症发生率最低。

The long-term outcomes, up to 18 months, of adolescents whose family had died by suicide suggest the incidence of major depressive disorder is higher in those who had depression before the family's suicide, intermediate in those who developed depression immediately after the suicide, and lowest in those who were not depressed immediately after the suicide.

那些在亲人死后变得抑郁的青少年表现更接近于自杀死亡的亲人，他们表现出更强烈的悲伤感，并且更加容易发生自杀。在亲人自杀的6年内，有创伤性悲伤症状的青少年比没有创伤性悲伤的青少年报告自杀意念的可能性高5倍。

Those who became depressed after the death were closer to the family who died by suicide, showed more intense grief, and had more intense exposure to the suicide. Within 6 years of the suicide of a family, adolescents with syndromal levels of traumatic grief were 5 times more likely to report suicidal ideation than those without traumatic grief.

然而，经历亲人自杀死亡的青少年的自杀发生率并不高于那些不知道身边亲人死于自杀的青少年。自杀死亡的青少年，其兄弟姐妹在6个月内发生抑郁障碍的风险增加7倍。

However, there was no greater incidence of suicide attempts among adolescents with a family who had died by suicide than among adolescents who did not know someone who died by suicide. Adolescent siblings of youths who died by suicide had a sevenfold increased risk for developing major depressive disorder within 6 months.

然而，一项关于对因自杀死亡的青少年的兄弟姐妹进行的3年随访研究发现，其兄弟姐妹比其朋友更为悲痛，但随访中其兄弟姐妹和朋友的精神障碍发生率与那些没有朋友或兄弟姐妹死于自杀的青少年差别不大。

However, in a related 3-year follow-up of siblings of adolescents who died by suicide, the siblings suffered more significant grief than the friends of the adolescents who died by suicide, although the rates of psychiatric disorders in follow-up were similar to those for adolescents who did not have a friend or sibling who died by suicide.

这些研究表明，在亲属自杀后，精神症状和功能受损的风险将增加。因此，应在患者死亡后不久向家庭成员提供精神心理干预，并坚持保持干预以降低精神障碍的发生风险，这种干预对于青少年以及目睹自杀或死亡现场的人尤为重要。

These studies suggest an increased risk of psychiatric symptoms and impairment after the suicide of a relative. As a result, psychiatric intervention should be offered to family members shortly after the death and maintained to reduce risk for psychiatric impairment. Such intervention is particularly important for youths and for those who witnessed the suicide or were at the scene of the death.

精神心理干预的目标包括识别和治疗重度抑郁和创伤后应激障碍及其相关症状。对亲属或朋友自杀后的青少年应进行长期随访评估和干预，以降低复发性抑郁症和其他疾病的风险。

The goals of psychiatric intervention include the identification and treatment of major depressive and post-traumatic stress disorders as well as related symptoms. Longer-term follow-up with evaluation and intervention for adolescents bereaved after the suicide of a relative or friend is also indicated to decrease the risk for recurrent depression and other morbidities.

对于那些在青少年自杀后丧失亲人的家庭成员，需要采用家庭评估和干预。尤其是与自杀者情感联系较深的青少年，悲伤的评估和治疗对于降低青少年自杀意念的风险可能同样重要。对于自杀者的所有家庭成员和亲密朋友，应该将他们转介给相关组织以寻求支持。

Furthermore, a family approach to evaluation and intervention is needed for those who are bereaved after an adolescent's suicide. Evaluation and treatment of grief may be similarly important in reducing risk for suicidal ideation among youths who are bereaved as a result of the suicide of a person who is emotionally important to them. For all family members and close friends of individuals who die by suicide, referral to a survivor support group can be helpful.

3.2.8 其他简要干预

3.2.8 Other Brief Interventions

(1)快速转介。

(1)Rapid Referral.

快速转介干预即在出院后七天内(最好在出院后 24 小时内)为患者提供的随访预约。与门诊医护人员协同制定转诊协议有助于快速转介。在选择转介推荐时，需考虑患者的需求并解决患者门诊就诊的相关困难。

The Rapid Referral intervention involves obtaining a follow-up appointment for the patient that occurs within seven days of discharge—ideally, within 24 hours of discharge. Developing referral agreements with outpatient providers may facilitate this process. Consider the patient's needs and troubleshoot barriers to accessing outpatient services when choosing a referral.

实施步骤：

①制定社区资源清单,医务人员可以使用该清单与门诊医生进行转诊预约,尤其是擅长自杀评估、管理和治疗的医生。

②征得患者同意后向转诊的医生提供患者急诊科就诊的临床信息。

③在患者出院前,联系门诊医生,在患者出院后一周内安排优先门诊预约。

④对于在非工作时间内到医院就诊的患者,确定其他值班医师为其安排时间完成随访。

⑤如果无法在出院后一周内安排第一次随访预约,请考虑以下选项:

• 请患者与初级保健提供者(PCP)进行随访预约。在患者许可的情况下,联系 PCP 讨论患者的病情和转诊原因。大多数 PCP 很少意识到患者的自杀意念或自杀企图。寻求帮助以确保患者能接受门诊心理健康治疗。

• 制定与当地危机干预中心合作的流程,为这些患者提供随访支持。一些危机中心会与最近从急诊科出院的患者建立随访联系,以保障治疗的连续性和提供其他帮助。另外,危机中心服务是免费向公众开放的。

⑥使用社区资源清单中的信息解决患者接受治疗的困难(例如,没有健康保险或交通问题)。

Action Steps:

①Develop a community resource list that personnel can use for making referral appointments to outpatient providers. Highlight providers who are skilled in suicide assessment, management, and treatment.

② Request the patient's consent to provide clinical information about the ED visit to the referral provider.

③Before the patient is discharged, call an outpatient provider to schedule an urgent outpatient appointment for a date within a week of discharge.

④For patients who present to the hospital during off-hours, identify other personnel to schedule the follow-up appointment during regular business hours.

⑤If unable to schedule the first follow-up appointment for a date within a week of discharge, consider these options:

• Refer the patient for a follow-up appointment with a primary care provider (PCP). With the patient's permission, contact the PCP to discuss the patient's condition and reason for the referral. Most PCPs are not aware of their patients' suicidal ideation or attempts. Ask for help in securing outpatient mental health treatment.

• Develop a protocol for working with a local crisis center to provide follow-up support for these patients. Some crisis centers make follow-up contacts with patients who have recently been discharged from EDs to facilitate linkages to care and provide additional support. And crisis center services are free and open to the public.

⑥ Troubleshoot the patient's access-to-care barriers (e.g., lack of health insurance or transportation) using information from the community resources list.

（2）关怀联络。

（2）Caring Contacts.

关怀联络是指在患者出院后保持与患者简短的沟通。它们可以由医护人员或其他医务人员提供，可以是一次或多次的沟通，也可以是单向或双向的沟通。这些沟通旨在加强患者对出院后治疗计划的依从性，同时通过表达对患者的持续关心以加强与患者的联络。对于无法到门诊治疗或不愿意接受门诊治疗的患者，关怀联络可能尤其必要。

Caring contacts are brief communications with the patient after discharge from the hospital. They may be made by the department provider or other personnel, be one-time or recurring contacts, and involve one-way or two-way communication. These contacts are meant to facilitate adherence to the discharge plan and promote a feeling of connectedness by demonstrating continued interest in the patient. Caring contacts may be especially helpful for patients who have barriers to outpatient care or are unwilling to access this care.

实施步骤：

①通过明信片、信件、电子邮件、短信或电话对出院患者进行随访。这些联系可以由临床工作者或急诊科非医疗人员进行，亦可通过电脑完成。电话随访则需要培训。

②使用自动化系统提供关怀性联络，例如邮寄或通过电子邮件发送的明信片或短信。一些电子健康记录系统也可以完成这些任务。

③考虑与当地危机中心达成协议，允许其工作人员与最近出院的病人建立关怀联络。

Action Steps：

① Follow up with discharged patients via postcards, letters, e-mail, text messages, or phone calls. These contacts can be made by clinical staff or non-medical ED personnel and may be automated. Phone calls will require training.

② Use automated systems to provide caring contacts, such as mailing or e-mailing postcards or text messages. Some electronic health record systems can perform these functions.

③ Consider establishing an agreement with a local crisis center that allows its staff to make caring contacts with recently discharged patients.

3.3 患者的社会支持网络

3.3 Social Support Networks for Patients

社会支持通常被认为是稳固的关系和良好的心理健康的关键组成部分,但它究竟意味着什么？从本质上讲,社会支持包括拥有一个你可以在需要的时候求助的包含家人和朋友的人际网络。无论你正面临个人危机,需要立即帮助,还是你只是想花时间和关心你的人在一起,这些关系在你的日常生活中扮演着重要的角色。

Social support is often identified as a key component of solid relationships and strong psychological health, but what exactly does it mean? Essentially, social support involves a network of family and friends that you can turn to in times of need. Whether you are facing a personal crisis and need immediate assistance, or you just want to spend time with people who care about you, these relationships play a critical role in how you function in your day-to-day life.

正是社会支持在人们面临压力的时候帮助他们振作起来,并常常给予他们继续前进和快速成长的力量。但社会支持肯定不是一条单行道,除了依靠别人,你还可以给生活中许多人支持。

It is social support that builds people up during times of stress and often gives them the strength to carry on and even thrive. But social support is certainly not a one-way street. In addition to relying on others, you also serve as a form of support for many people in your life.

社会支持是个人应对压力时社会网络提供的心理和物质资源。这种社会支持可以不同的形式出现。有时,它可能是当一个人在生病时帮助其完成各种日常工作,或在他们需要时提供经济援助。

Social support refers to the psychological and material resources provided by a social network to help individuals cope with stress. Such social support may come in different forms. Sometimes it might involve helping a person with various daily tasks when they are ill or offering financial assistance when they are in need.

在其他情况下,当朋友们面临困难的时候,你可以给他们一些建议。有时,它可能只是简单的照料、同情和对亲人的关切。

In other situations, it could involve giving advice to a friend when they are facing a difficult situation. And sometimes it simply involves providing caring, empathy, and concern for loved ones in need.

多项研究表明,社会支持是降低自杀风险的保护性因素。社会支持通常被定义为一种信念,即一个人被关心并能得到帮助。然而,社会支持是一个包括多个维度的宽泛概念,不同的学者对社会支持的定义也不尽相同,包括社会支持的来源(例如家人和朋友)、支持对个人的意义、支持的数量和质量等。

Multiple studies have identified social support as a protective factor in reducing suicidality. Social support is generally defined as the belief that one is cared about and has available assistance. However, social support is a broad construct consisting of multiple dimensions, and various authors have conceptualized social support differently, including whom the social support comes from (i.e., family and friends), the personal meaning derived from the supports, and the quantity and quality of the supports.

这些不同的维度似乎都与心理健康预后有着独特的关系。社会支持以及与家庭成员和朋友频繁而积极的互动有助于产生归属感,这是社会融合的一个指标。相反,缺乏社会支持、不频繁的社会互动和频繁的消极互动(被认为是不愉快的、漠不关心的行为或破坏正常关系的行为,如批评和过多的要求)会导致归属感受挫,或不能满足归属的需求。

These diverse dimensions appear to have unique relationships with mental health outcomes. Social support and frequent and positive interactions with family members and friends contribute to a sense of belonging, which is an indicator of social integration. In contrast, lack of social support, infrequent social interactions, and frequent negative interactions (behaviors that are perceived as unpleasant, insensitive, or violations of relationship norms, such as criticism and excessive demands) result in thwarted belongingness, or an unmet need to belong.

自杀的人际理论认为归属感是自杀的保护性因素。具体来讲,良好的归属感能减少自杀,而受挫的归属感可能成为自杀的危险因素。归属感源于社会支持,包括家庭支持或朋友间的联络等,研究表明归属感与自杀意念和自杀企图呈负相关。

The interpersonal theory of suicide posits that a sense of belonging is an instrumental factor in suicidality. More specifically, belongingness is protective against suicidality, whereas thwarted belongingness is a risky factor for suicidality. Belongingness comes from social support, including family support or connections between friends and so on. Research has indicated that belongingness is inversely associated with suicide ideation and attempts.

在不同类型的社会支持中，家庭支持通常是影响患者适应疾病最重要的因素之一。一个支持性的家庭环境可以保护个人免受疾病带来的潜在精神病理影响。

Among the different types of social support, family support is generally one of the most important factors affecting how patients adapt to illness. The perception of a supportive family environment may protect individuals from the potential psychopathological effects stemming from the physical impact of their disease.

此外，在生病时，家庭往往是主要的支持来源，无论是通过实质性的支持（如做饭和喂药），还是情感上的支持。在癌症和终末期疾病患者中，较高的家庭支持水平与较低抑郁水平相关，而家庭支持缺乏与慢性疾病患者的自杀率相关。

Moreover, family is frequently the main source of support in times of illness, whether through tangible instrumental support, such as preparing meals and administering medication, or through emotional support. In cancer and end-stage disease patients, higher levels of family support are associated with lower levels of depression, while lack of family support has been linked with increased suicide rates in chronic disease patients.

研究发现，能被感知的家庭支持作为一种综合概念是抑郁症和自杀意念的主要保护因素。事实上，低家庭支持患者较高家庭支持患者的抑郁障碍发生率高5倍以上，而自杀意念高4倍。

Among the central findings of certain studies, perceived family support as a composite construct emerges as a major correlate of both depression and suicidal ideation. Indeed, those participants reporting the highest level of perceived family support were over five times less likely than those at the lowest level to register BDI-IA-defined depression and four times less likely to endorse suicidal ideation.

部分研究发现同伴的支持和父母的支持都与自杀意念的显著降低相关。然而，父母的社会支持可以改善抑郁和自杀意念之间的关系，而同伴的社会支持可以改善进食障碍症状和自杀意念之间的关系。

Some studies found that both peer support and parental support were significantly associated with reduced suicide ideation. However, parental social support moderated the relationship between depression and suicide ideation, while peer social support moderated the relationship between eating disorder symptoms and suicide ideation.

其他研究进一步发现，来自家庭的社会支持可显著减少自杀意念，但是来自其他重要的人和朋友的社会支持对自杀意念无显著性影响。这些研究进一步强调了社会支持来源的重要性,家庭支持在减少自杀意念方面可能尤其重要。

Other studies have found further that perceived social support from family had a significant effect in reducing suicide ideation, but social support from significant others and friends was not statistically significant. These studies furthered the importance of measuring the source of the social support, as family support may be particularly important in reducing suicide ideation.

总的来说,与朋友和家人接触的频率越高,主观的家庭亲密程度越高,自杀意念和自杀尝试行为的发生率就越低。一个严重的挑战或威胁如自杀行为,往往与社会支持网络的变化有关。

On the whole, more frequent contact with friends and family, and higher levels of subjective family closeness are associated with lower rates of suicide ideation and attempts. A serious challenge or threat, such as suicidal behaviors, is accompanied by a mobilization of the social network.

在这种情况下,朋友与家人在自杀行为发生后,可能需要联合起来为患者提供更多的帮助。另外,那些曾经想过或试图自杀的恢复期患者更可能向朋友或家人求助,以预防未来的自杀行为,或调动支持资源来应对持续的心理应激。

In this case, friends and family may rally to provide increased assistance in the wake of suicidal behaviors. Alternatively, respondents who have previously thought about or attempted suicide may be more likely to turn to friends and family to prevent future suicidal behaviors or marshal support resources in coping with ongoing stressors.

4 自杀风险患者的随访

4 Follow-up of Patients at Risk of Suicide

4.1 出院计划清单
4.1 Discharge Planning Checklist

出院计划提供了将有自杀风险的患者与后续护理资源联系起来的关键机会。精心设计的出院计划可以改善从医院到社区的过渡,减少再入院率并提高患者满意度。

Discharge planning provides an important opportunity to link patients with suicide risk to sources of follow-up care. Well-conceived discharge planning can improve transitions from hospital to community, reduce readmissions, and increase patient satisfaction.

有自杀风险的患者在获得后续护理的过程中可能面临着多重障碍,包括财务问题、保险未能涵盖之处、交通问题、耻辱感、日程安排冲突以及社区治疗能力有限等。通过让患者及其支持系统作为同伴参与制定出院计划可以预测和解决障碍问题。

Patients with suicide risk may face multiple barriers to getting follow-up care, including financial problems, insurance coverage gaps, lack of transportation, stigma, scheduling conflicts, and limited treatment capacity in the community. Anticipate and troubleshoot problems by involving the patient and his or her support system as partners in the discharge planning process.

对有自杀风险的患者使用出院计划清单。清单中的项目可以纳入所在医疗机构现有的出院计划协议和电子健康记录系统。

Use the discharge planning checklist with patients with suicide risk. Items in the checklist may be incorporated into your facility's existing discharge planning protocols and electronic health record system.

清单宜强调自杀风险患者出院计划中的以下9项最佳实践,一些项目也出现在基于急诊科的简要自杀预防干预措施中。可根据所在医疗机构的人员结构、可获得资源和患者需求来调整清单。

The checklist should highlight the 9 best practices for planning the discharge of patients with suicide risk. Some items also appear in the ED-based brief suicide prevention interventions. The checklist may be adapted according to the staffing structures, available resources, and needs of the patients in your medical setting.

（1）让患者作为同伴参与进来。

医务人员尽可能采用激励性谈话技巧,鼓励患者关注生活的积极方面,寻找自杀的保护因素,与患者家人和朋友共同努力,帮助患者顺利恢复。例如询问患者"出院回家对你而言将是什么样子?""生活中你最喜欢什么?"

（1）Involve the patient as a partner.

Medical staff should employ motivational conversation techniques as far as possible to encourage patients to focus on positive aspects of life, look for protective factors of suicide, and work with their families and friends to help them recover smoothly. Sample questions to ask include "What will being home be like for you?" and "What do you like most about your life?"

教会患者回归生活、融入生活。例如:"您可能还需要一点时间才能再次感到舒适,但您可以做的就是回到您的日常生活中,合理饮食、适当运动、规律睡眠、调整心态、积极应对。找到一个自己的喜好或者最喜欢的消遣方式,例如听音乐、看电影或者收集东西,以平稳心境并保持积极。尽可能多地与他人进行互动,这会让您感受到被周围人支持、关心、需要和认可,并获得持久价值感"。

Teach patients to return to life and integrate into life. For example, "it may take you a little time to feel comfortable again, but what you can do is to go back to your daily life, eat properly, exercise properly, sleep regularly, adjust your mind and be active. Find a hobby or favorite pastime, such as listening to music, watching movies or collecting things to calm your mind and make it positive. Engage in interactive activities with others as much as possible. This will allow you to feel supported, cared for, needed, validated by those around you and gain a sense of lasting value."

告诉患者家属"和谐的家庭氛围以及亲密的人际关系可以预防患者再次自杀,缓和家庭成员的关系。在生活中要真诚地关心与理解患者,多陪伴他,减轻孤独感,倾听患者的想法、感受和愿望。"

Tell the patient's family that "a harmonious family atmosphere and close interpersonal relationship can prevent the patient from committing suicide again and ease the relationship between family members. Sincerely care and understand the patient in life, spend more time with him/her, reduce loneliness, and listen to his/her thoughts, feelings and wishes."

（2）落实预约随访。

在患者出院后7天内，最好是24小时内，与精神保健人员、初级保健人员或者其他门诊卫生服务人员联系，安排紧急预约随访。如果患者出院前不能安排预约随访时间，强烈建议患者在回家前几天寻求随访治疗。

（2）Make follow-up appointments.

Schedule an urgent follow-up appointment (when feasible within seven days of discharge; ideally within 24 hours) with a mental health care provider, primary care provider, or other outpatient provider. If the patients cannot schedule follow-up appointments before discharge, it is strongly recommended that they seek follow-up care a few days before returning home.

如果无法预约门诊卫生服务，请在常规工作时间内计划第二次预约，或留言请求优先安排该患者。如果这些方法无法实现，可以在患者允许的情况下，找一位值得信赖的护理人员或同行专家帮助安排预约。同时提醒您的患者，当他再次产生自杀想法或当地医疗团队无法提供所需护理时，急诊科一年365天每天24小时开放。

If the outpatient provider is unavailable, plan for a second call during regular working hours or leave a message requesting priority scheduling for the patient. If these steps fail, and with the patient's permission, enlist a trusted caregiver or peer specialist to help schedule the appointment. Remind your patient that the emergency department is open 24 hours a day, 365 days a year, when he or she is experiencing suicidal thought or when the local medical team is unable to provide the care needed.

（3）审查并讨论患者的出院计划。

口头审查患者出院计划，包括审查药物、患者自杀的危险信号、内部应对策略、分散危机负面影响的方法、可提供支持的家人或朋友、可联络给予帮助的专业人员或机构、保障环境安全的方法。安全计划可用于解决患者护理计划中与自杀风险有关的要素。

（3）Review and discuss the patient care plan.

Verbally review the patient care plan, including a review of medications, the patient's individual warning signs, internal coping strategies, ways to distract oneself from the crisis, the family members or friends who can provide support, professionals and agencies to contact for help and ways to make the environment safe. A safety plan may be used to address elements of the patient care plan related to suicide risk.

（4）讨论障碍因素和解决方案。

讨论自杀风险患者在遵循出院计划时的潜在障碍,例如保险问题、交通问题、羞耻感、日程安排冲突等,确定可能的解决途径或者替代办法。鼓励患者及其支持系统作为同伴参与出院计划的制定,例如询问患者"缺乏健康保险怎么办?""后续护理由谁完成? 在哪儿实施? 什么时候实施?""最近的心理门诊距离您家有十公里远,您将乘坐什么交通工具去?""您的家人中谁能陪同您去接受后续治疗?"全面的考量和预测问题,有助于患者顺利接受后续护理。

（4）Discuss barriers and resolutions.

Discuss potential barriers (lack of health insurance, transportation problems, stigma, scheduling conflicts, *et al*) to following the patient care plan and identify possible solutions or alternatives. Encourage the patients and their support systems to participate as partners in the development of discharge plans, such as asking the patients "what about the lack of health insurance?" "Who does the follow-up care? Where is it implemented? When will it be implemented?" "The nearest psychological clinic is ten kilometers away from your home. What transportation will you take?" "Who in your family can accompany you to follow-up treatment?" Comprehensive consideration and prediction of problems can contribute to receiving follow-up care smoothly.

（5）提供危机中心的电话号码。

为患者提供当地危机热线或国家预防自杀生命线电话号码。危机中心,也称为自杀热线或求助热线,可以作为医疗机构的合作伙伴来照顾有自杀风险的患者。他们提供全周全天候的保密服务,包括评估和转介,并不向个人收取任何费用。

（5）Provide a crisis center phone number.

Provide the patient with the phone number of a local crisis hotline or the National Suicide Prevention Lifeline. Crisis centers, also referred to as suicide hotlines or helplines, can be partners to medical settings in caring for patients with suicide risk. They provide confidential services 24/7, including assessment and referrals, at no cost to the individual.

国家预防自杀生命线的危机中心成员遵循评估自杀风险和紧急风险的最佳实践,并有机会获得全国危机中心的同行和资源网络。一些危机热线为许多不同的语言提供翻译,根据您所在地区的语言群体,您可以找到为这些群体提供危机服务的当地合作伙伴。

Crisis center members of the National Suicide Prevention Lifeline (NSPL) follow best practices in assessing suicide risk and imminent risk and have access to a national network of crisis center peers and resources. Some crisis lines provide translation for a number of different languages; based on the linguistic groups in your area, you may be able to find local partners who provide crisis services to these groups.

联合委员会和国家预防自杀战略建议,每位有自杀风险的患者在出院前都会以书面形式收到附近危机中心的电话号码。医院也可考虑与危机中心签订正式协议,为这些患者提供随访服务。例如,医院可以征得患者同意,让危机中心以电话的形式提供后续支持。

The Joint Commission and the National Strategy for Suicide Prevention recommend that every patient with suicide risk be handed written information with the phone number of the nearest crisis center before discharge. Hospitals may also consider making formal agreements with crisis centers to provide follow-up services for these patients. For example, the hospital may obtain patient consent for the crisis center to provide follow-up support in the form of phone calls.

这些服务对难以获取门诊心理健康服务的患者特别有用。与患者达成协议,当其再次萌发自杀意念时,必须立即与当地危机中心或者医院工作人员联系,并寻求帮助。医务人员可以告诉患者:"您的健康是宝贵的,我们衷心希望您可以照顾并享受您的健康,当您遇到困难时,请不要犹豫,联系我们,我们始终与您同在!"

These services can be particularly helpful for patients with barriers to accessing outpatient mental health services. Reach an agreement with the patient that when he or she has suicidal ideation again, he or she must contact the staff of the local crisis center or the hospital and ask for help at once. Medical staff can tell patients "Your health is precious, and we earnestly hope that you will take care of it and enjoy it. When you are in trouble, please do not hesitate to contact us. We are always with you!"

(6) 讨论限制致命手段的途径。

首先,告诉患者及其家属自杀风险有时会迅速增加,因此这期间限制致命手段至关重要。其次,询问患者及其家属是否有机会获取致命手段。如果有,询问具体位置。然后,对报告有机会获取致命手段的患者提供适当的咨询。

(6) Discuss limiting access to lethal means.

First, tell patients and their families that the risk of suicide sometimes increases rapidly which makes it crucial to limit lethal means during this time. Second, ask patients and their families if they have access to lethal means. If the patient has access to firearms, ask about the location. Then provide appropriate counseling to the patients who report having access to lethal means.

最后,确定限制获得致命性手段的策略,例如在自杀危险消失之前将农药存放在朋友家中,并允许家人将药物锁起来并保管钥匙,在必要时分配药物以防止患者服毒。例如,"我不知道您家里是否有农药,但如果有,请将它存放在远离家的地方或者将其锁起来并让你信任的人保管钥匙,这样对您来说更安全。"

Finally identify strategies for limiting access to lethal means, such as storing farm chemicals at a friend's house until the suicidal crisis has passed, and allowing a family member to keep medications under lock and key and dispense them as necessary in order to prevent self-poisoning. Sample expressions include "I don't know whether you have farm chemicals in your house, but if you do, it's safe for you to store it far away from home or lock it up and have someone you trust keep the key."

(7)提供书面说明和教育材料。

向患者提供其出院计划的书面版本以及有关其健康状况和治疗建议的教育资源(如安全计划指南、降低自杀风险的安全计划治疗手册、社区资源清单)。提供有关患者病情恶化时该如何处理的信息,包括返回医疗机构复诊的时间。

(7) Provide written instructions and education materials.

Give the patient a written version of the patient care plan and educational resources (e.g., safety plan guide, safety plan treatment manual to reduce suicide risk, community resource list) about his or her condition and treatment recommendations. Provide information on what to do if the patient's condition worsens, including when to return to the medical setting.

当您频繁产生自杀意念或反复睡眠障碍,您应当请家人或朋友保护您的安全,消除获取致命性手段的途径,并且最好及时寻求心理健康干预。

When you frequently arise suicidal ideation or recurrent sleep disorders, you should ask your family member or friends to protect your safety, eliminating access to lethal means. It would be best to seek mental health intervention in time.

(8)向转诊卫生服务提供者共享患者健康信息。

患者带着自杀风险进入新的治疗机构,如果转诊接收者对患者病情了解不全面,未及时采取有效的自杀预防措施,那么患者很有可能会再次自杀,甚至自杀死亡。因此,要征得患者的同意,以便与转诊卫生服务提供者共享他或她的健康信息。向转诊卫生服务提供者发送患者出院小结,以保持护理的连续性,帮助转诊服务提供者做出明智的决策。

(8) Share patient health information with referral providers.

When a patient with the risk of suicide enter new treatment institutions, if the referral recipient does not fully understand the patient's condition and fails to take effective suicide prevention measures in time, the patient is likely to commit suicide again or even die by suicide. Therefore obtain the patient's consent for sharing his or her health information with referral providers. Send the referral provider a copy of the patient's discharge summary to keep continuity of care and help referral providers make informed decisions.

(9) 关怀性沟通和照顾。

卫生保健人员应当关心和关注患者,尊重患者的隐私,与患者沟通,向患者传达药物治疗和心理治疗是有效的,鼓励其遵从护理计划。与患者确定随访方案,如明信片、信件、电子邮件、短信或者电话,及时疏导患者的负性情绪,不断灌输信心和希望。

(9) Communicate care and concern.

Health care providers should show care and concern, respect patients' privacy, communicate with patients, convey the information that medications and psychotherapy are effective, and encourage patients to follow their patient care plans. Determine with patients their follow-up schemes, such as postcards, letters, e-mails, text messages or phone calls, timely release the negative emotions of the patient, and continuously instill confidence and hope.

介绍自己时要有眼神交流并与每个人握手。让患者在不被中断的情况下说话一分钟——这可以提高患者的满意度,并且还可以获得在平时询问中可能遗漏的信息。

Make eye contact and shake hands with everyone as you introduce yourself. Let the patient talk for a minute without interruption—it increases his/her satisfaction and you'll also get information you otherwise might have missed in your usual questioning.

附:给门诊精神健康提供者的信函样本

Attached:Sample Letter to Outpatient Mental Health Providers

日期 Date

姓名 Name

地址 Address

您好[心理健康专业名称]：

我们[以医疗机构的名义]正在对我们的科室进行改革，以帮助我们更好地识别和治疗自杀风险较高的患者。我们正在培训我们的工作人员，以更好地识别常见的自杀警告信号，并筛查患者的自杀意念。随着我们对自杀风险的警惕加强，我们想探讨如何与您合作，以提高我们医院出院的自杀风险患者的连续性护理。

Dear [Mental Health Professional Name]:

We [in the name of the medical institution] are implementing changes in our department to help us better identify and treat patients who are at elevated risk for suicide. We are training our staff to better recognize the common warning signs of suicide and to screen patients for suicidal ideation. As we step up our vigilance for suicide risk, we would like to explore how we might partner with you to improve continuity of care for our patients with suicide risk who are discharged.

我们愿意与您合作，以确保我们的患者能够获得贵机构的专业知识和技术。由于合作照顾需要有效的沟通，我建议我们通过会议或电话来分享观点，并开发合作模式。我们还想探讨制定转诊方案的可行性，该方案将促进自杀风险患者在出院后7天内获得后续护理。我们将在不久的将来联系您来探索这种可能性。

您真诚的伙伴×××

We would like to work with you to assure the best access for our patients to your specialized knowledge and expertise. Since collaborative care requires strong communication, I would like to propose that we set up a meeting or phone call to share perspectives and develop a model for collaboration. I would also like to explore the feasibility of developing a referral protocol that would facilitate access to follow-up care within seven days of discharge for patients with suicide risk. I will be contacting your office in the near future to explore this possibility.

Sincerely yours.

患者自杀风险管理指导手册（汉英对照）

160

4.2 社区资源清单模板

4.2 Community Resource List Template

社区资源清单可以在当地社区促进转诊卫生服务提供者提供服务。此模板可用于开发完整的本地清单。开始使用时，请咨询可能有现有清单的社区人力服务机构。每年更新此清单以保持准确性。

Community resource lists can facilitate making referrals to services in the local community. This template may be used to develop a complete local list. To get started，consult with a community human services agency that may have an existing list to share. Update this list annually to maintain accuracy.

卫生保健、精神卫生和药物滥用资源

社区精神健康机构	社区健康中心
私人实践心理健康提供者	私人实践初级护理提供者
心理健康危机服务	部落健康/传统治疗师
同伴支持服务（如 NAMI、健康中心）	医疗保险连接器
VA 自杀预防协调员	VA 诊所
药物滥用治疗	艾滋病毒/艾滋病信息和测试地点
匿名戒酒会/匿名毒瘾者互助会	糖尿病的预防和支持
医院/紧急服务	急救医务组
儿童/青少年精神科诊所	其他

其他资源

911/211服务信息	儿童事务处/社会服务
紧急庇护所	儿童护理转介
房屋服务	家长培训/长者/健康及健康中心
青少年庇护所/安全之家	家长热线
LGBT 服务	运输供应者
家庭暴力服务	高级服务
家庭暴力热线	社区项目
宗教/精神支持	自助小组/祈祷小屋/谈话圈
法律援助/法律救助/部落法庭	粮食银行
WIC 和/或印度健康服务营养	学校学生服务/部落教育部门
职业培训/就业计划	其他
ESL 服务	其他

Health care, mental health, and substance abuse resources

Community mental health agencies	Community health centers
Private practice mental health	Private practice primary care providers
Mental health crisis services	Tribal health/Traditional healers
Peer support services(e.g.,NAMI, Wellness centers)	Health insurance connector
VA suicide prevention coordinator	VA clinic
Substance abuse treatment	HIV/AIDS information and testing sites
Alcoholics anonymous/narcotics anonymous	Diabetes prevention and support
Hospital /emergency services	Paramedic emergency medical services unit
Children/youth psychiatric clinic	other

Others resources

911/211 Information services	Children's services office/social services
Emergency shelter	Child care referrals
Housing services	Parent training/elder/health and wellness
Youth shelter/safe house	Parent helpline
LGBT Services	Transportation providers
Domestic violence services	Senior services
Domestic violence helpline	Community programs
Religious/Spiritual support	Self-help groups/prayers lodges/Talking Circles
Legal assistance/Legal aid/Tribal courts	Food bank
WIC and/or Indian services nutrition	School student services/tribal education department
Job training and placement programs	Other
ESL Services	Other

中国危机干预电话

中国心理危机与自杀干预中心救助热线:010－62715275

北京心理援助热线:010－82951332、800－810－1117(24小时面向全球提供中文服务的免费危机干预热线)

北京红枫妇女热线:010－64073800(周一至周五 9:00－18:00)

中科院心理所咨询志愿者热线:010－64851106

北京协和启迪心理咨询中心救助热线:010－65132928

北京1980阳光部落心理咨询热线:010-68001980

上海市危机干预中心:021-64383562

上海林紫心理咨询中心:021-64333183,64333512

广州市青少年心理健康热线:020-83182110

广州市心理危机干预中心热线:020-81899120(24小时)

南京生命求助热线:(025)86528082

南京自杀干预中心救助热线:16896123(24小时)

杭州心理研究与干预中心救助热线:(0571)85029595(24小时)

武汉市精神卫生中心咨询热线:(027)85844666(8:00-21:00)/ 51826188

深圳心理危机干预热线(康宁医院):(0755)25629459

天津市心理危机干预热线:(022)96051199

四川省心理危机干预中心热线:(028)87577510 / 87528604

湖南省《法制周报》心理危机干预中心热线:(0731)4839110

重庆市心理危机干预中心热线:(023)66644499

青岛市心理危机干预中心自杀干预热线:(0532)85669120(24小时)/ 86669120(8:30-11:00;13:30-16:00)

石家庄心理危机干预热线:(0311)6799116

苏州西园寺观世音心理疏导热线:(0512)65833539(每周二、四、六19:00-21:00)

长春市心理援助热线:(0431)86985000(24小时)、(0431)86985333(8:00-16:00)

香港地区生命热线:(+852)23820000

香港地区撒玛利亚热线:(+852)28960000

5 自杀风险患者的文书记录
5 Documentation of Suicide Risk Patients

5.1 记录就诊过程

5.1 Record the Course of Treatment

全面记录为自杀风险患者提供的护理可以提高护理质量,同时可以证明医疗服务提供者和医院为达到国家护理标准所做的努力。假设为患者提供了高质量的、以患者为中心的护理,完整的文件是预防和解决与护理这些患者相关的潜在法律问题的关键因素。

Fully documenting the care provided for patients with suicide risk improves quality of care and can demonstrate provider and hospital efforts to meet national care standards. Assuming that patients are provided with high-quality, patient-centered care, full documentation is the key factor for preventing and addressing potential legal problems related to caring for these patients.

决策过程中的每个步骤,以及与患者、家庭成员、其他重要人员、其他照顾者的所有沟通应予以记录。卫生服务提供者还可以考虑将这些和其他自杀预防数据要素纳入医院电子病历和实践管理系统,以促进文件处理过程。

Every step in the decision-making process and all communication with the patient, his or her family members and significant others, and other caregivers should be recorded. Providers may also consider ways to embed these and other suicide prevention data elements into hospital electronic medical records and practice management systems to facilitate the documentation process.

行动步骤:在记录患者及其探视相关的信息时,请指明您已查阅或试图查阅之前与患者进行过互动的其他卫生服务提供者的记录。使用描述性的术语,表明您可以从其他人的轮班中识别患者,使用非评判性的术语,并包含引号(例如,"我不是自杀的")。

Action steps: When documenting information about the patient and his or her visit, indicate that you reviewed or attempted to review the records from other providers who interacted with the patient before you. Use descriptive terms to show that you can identify the patient from among others seen in that shift. Use nonjudgmental terms, and include quotes (e.g., "I'm not suicidal").

记录的具体内容：

• 患者如何来到医院（如"开车""由家人带来"）；

• 患者就诊的具体原因，以明确的方式说明（如"探访护士关注死亡的提法"，而不是"精神分裂症"）；

• 患者对所发生事情的叙述——来访的原因；

• 与患者家属、支持者、之前的卫生服务提供者及门诊服务提供者进行沟通或尝试沟通；

• 提供了什么，包括获得心理健康咨询和简要的自杀预防干预；

• 实施筛查和评估，其结果包括决策支持工具与患者的危险因素和保护因素；

• 对入院或出院决定的主要考虑因素，包括考虑但拒绝任何决定或行动的原因；

• 患者用药信息；

• 现场提供的干预措施，包括简单的支持和解决问题的努力；

• 患者对治疗的明确偏好；

• 就诊期间遇到的任何挑战；

• 担忧以及为缓解这些问题而采取的行动；

• 评估患者获得致命手段和提供相关咨询；

• 患者出院护理计划或安全计划；

• 给出的转介类型，包括提供者的联系信息；

• 与患者的任何后续接触。

What to Document：

• How the patient arrived (e.g., "drove", "brought by family")；

• The specific reason for the patient's visit, stated in a clear way (e.g., "visiting nurse was concerned about a reference to death"; not, for example, "decompensating schizophrenic")；

• The patient's account of what happened—the reason for the visit；

• Communication or attempted communication with the patient's family, supports, previous providers, and outpatient providers；

• What was offered, including access to a mental health consultation and brief suicide prevention interventions；

• Screenings and assessments performed and their results, including the Decision Support Tool and the patient's risk and protective factors；

• Key considerations made for admission or discharge decisions, including the reasons why any decisions or actions were considered but rejected；

• Information about the patient's medications；

• Interventions provided onsite，including simple supportive and problem-solving efforts；

• The patient's stated preferences regarding treatment；

• Any challenges encountered during the visit；

• Concerns and actions taken to mitigate these concerns；

• Assessment of the patient's access to lethal means and provision of related counseling；

• Patient care plan for discharge or safety plan；

• Type of referral given，including provider contact information；

• Any subsequent contacts with the patient.

5.2 针对自杀问题的一般风险管理和文书管理

5.2 General Risk Management and Documentation Issues Specific to Suicide

风险管理是精神疾病治疗实践的重要组成部分,尤其是在有自杀风险患者的评估和管理方面。基于临床的风险管理是以患者为中心,支持治疗联盟和治疗过程。对于精神病医生最常见的诉讼、和解和判决问题是针对患者自杀。因此,当治疗有自杀行为的患者时,重要的是要意识到并关注某些一般风险管理注意事项。

Risk management is an important component of psychiatric practice，especially in the assessment and management of patients at risk for suicide. Clinical-based risk management is patient-centered and supports the therapeutic alliance and the treatment process. The most frequent lawsuits，settlements，and verdicts against psychiatrists are for patients' suicides. Thus，when treating a patient with suicidal behaviors，it is important to be aware of and pay attention to certain general risk management considerations.

患者医疗文件是医疗实践的基石,对风险管理也同样很重要。如果针对临床医生提出医疗事故索赔,自杀风险评估文件将协助法院评估在自杀风险患者治疗和管理中存在的许多临床复杂性和模糊性。

Documentation of patient care is a cornerstone of medical practice，but it is also essential to risk management. If a malpractice claim is brought against the clinicians，documentation of suicide risk assessments assists the court in evaluating the many clinical complexities and ambiguities that exist in the treatment and management of patients at suicide risk.

未记录自杀风险的评估和干预措施可能会使法院有理由断定医护没有做相应的处理。对于住院患者,记录住院治疗的风险评估方面也很重要,特别是在非自愿的情况下。因此,将自杀风险评估记录在病历中至关重要。

The failure to document suicide risk assessments and interventions may give the court reason to conclude they were not done. For patients who are hospitalized, it is also important to document the aspects of the risk assessment that justify inpatient treatment, particularly when it is occurring on an involuntary basis. Thus, it is crucial for the suicide risk assessment to be documented in the medical record.

尽管临床医生面临时间压力,但文档记录最好在自杀评估完成后马上完成。关于评估的原因(例如,复发、恶化、重大的生活事件)将作为患者自杀风险的评估背景。随后的讨论回顾了那些可能增加短期或长期自杀风险的因素以及展开评估的推理过程。还应注意临床结论和治疗计划的所有变化以及处理的依据。如果考虑其他干预措施或行动,但遭到拒绝,拒绝的理由也应记录。

Despite the time burdens faced by the clinicians, documentation is best done just after the suicide assessment is completed. Reference to the reason for the assessment (e.g., relapse, worsening, a reversal in the patient's life) will set the context for the evaluation. Subsequent discussion reviews the factors that may contribute to increased shorter-term or longer-term suicide risk as well as the reasoning process that went into the assessment. Clinical conclusions and any changes in the treatment plan should also be noted, along with the rationale for such actions. If other interventions or actions were considered but rejected, that reasoning should be recorded as well.

考虑一例患者在先前因自杀未遂住院治疗后处于缓解期,但最近复发的案例。精神科医生可能会记录自杀意念的存在,但是没有有关治疗计划或增加自杀风险的特定症状的证据(如激惹、重度焦虑、严重失眠)。患者承受的压力增加,并且处于某种痛苦中,但对支持有反应的情况也应记录。

Consider the example of a patient who was in remission after a prior hospitalization for a suicide attempt but recently had a relapse or a recurrent episode. The psychiatrist may document that suicidal ideation is present but there is no evidence of a specific plan or specific symptoms that would augment risk (i.e., agitation, severe anxiety, severe insomnia). It may also be noted that the patient is under increased stress and is in some distress but is responsive to support.

基于患者有接受帮助的意愿并且缺乏急性自杀危险因素的证据,持续性的门诊管理可能是合理的,同时调整治疗计划,例如增加就诊次数或者暂时增加抗焦虑药物剂量,或者与能提供支持的亲戚或朋友交谈以获取更多信息并巩固患者的支持系统。

On the basis of the patient's willingness to accept help and the lack of evidence of acute suicide risk factors, continued outpatient management may be reasonable, with changes in the treatment plan, such as increasing the frequency of visits, perhaps increasing anxiolytic medication doses temporarily, and perhaps talking with a supportive relative or friend to obtain more information and to solidify the patient's support system.

在所有医疗机构中,临床医生都应该意识到自杀风险评估是一个过程,而不仅仅是一个孤立的事件。在住院病房,评估记录的要点发生在入院、风险防范或观察水平变化、转科、通行证签发、患者病情变化和出院评估的时候。尤其是确定自杀预防水平(一对一监督或每15分钟检查一次等)应基于患者的临床表现,并得到临床证据的支持。

In all settings, the clinician should be aware that suicide risk assessment is a process and never simply an isolated event. On inpatient units, important points of documentation of assessment occur at admission, changes in the level of precautions or observations, transitions between treatment units, the issuance of passes, marked changes in the clinical condition of the patient, and evaluation for discharge. In particular, the determination of the level of suicide precautions (one-to-one versus every-15-minute checks, etc.) should be based on the patient's clinical presentation and be supported by a clinical rationale.

由于住院患者的治疗由一个多学科治疗团队提供,因此临床医生应该定期审阅患者的记录,或者在整个患者住院期间定期与团队成员进行口头沟通。在患者出院时,应记录继续住院和出院的风险—效益评估,并记录患者门诊治疗的随访安排。

Because care in inpatient settings is generally delivered by a multidisciplinary treatment team, it is important for the clinician either to review the patient's records regularly or to communicate verbally with staff throughout the patient's hospital stay. At the time of the patient's discharge from the hospital, risk-benefit assessments for both continued hospitalization and discharge should be documented, and follow-up arrangements for the patient's outpatient care should be recorded.

有关临床医生和患者之间良好协作、沟通和联盟的精心细致的文书包括以下内容:

• 风险评估;

- 记录决策过程；
- 治疗变化的描述；
- 与其他临床医生的沟通记录；
- 记录患者或家属的电话内容；
- 医嘱或者处方复印件；
- 既往治疗的病历（如果有），特别是与过去自杀企图有关的治疗。

Careful and Attentive Documentation about Good Collaboration, Communication, and Alliance between Clinician and Patient Including:

- Risk assessments;
- Record of decision-making processes;
- Descriptions of changes in treatment;
- Record of communications with other clinicians;
- Record of telephone calls from patients or family members;
- Prescription log or copies of actual prescriptions;
- Medical records of previous treatment, if available, particularly treatment related to past suicide attempts.

文书记录的关键时间点：

- 首次进行精神检查或入院；
- 发生任何自杀行为或想法；
- 每当有任何值得注意的临床变化时；
- 在增加特权或给予通行证之前以及在出院前，对移情和反移情问题进行监测，必要时应考虑二次意见。

Critical Junctures for Documentation:

- At first psychiatric assessment or admission;
- With occurrence of any suicidal behavior or ideation;
- Whenever there is any noteworthy clinical change;
- Before discharge, monitoring issues of transference and counter transference in order to optimize clinical judgment consultation; a second opinion being considered when necessary.

在门诊环境中，自杀风险评估和记录过程通常发生在初次访谈期间，在自杀意念、计划或行为出现或重新出现时，以及患者状况发生其他重大变化时。在这些时候适当地注意治疗计划的调整。对于精神分析或改良精神分析治疗的患者，精神科医生应遵循精神分析亚专科实践指南的推荐方案。

In outpatient settings, the process of suicide risk assessment and documentation typically occurs during the initial interview; at the emergence or reemergence of suicidal ideation, plans, or behaviors; and when there are other significant changes in the patient's condition. Revisions of the treatment plan are appropriately noted at these times. For patients in psychoanalysis or modified psychoanalytic treatment, the psychiatrist may elect to follow the charting recommendations of the psychoanalytic subspecialty practice guideline.

5.3 减轻责任担忧

5.3 Reducing Liability Concerns

照顾有自杀风险的患者可能会引发关于责任和伦理的问题和担忧。在医疗机构,可能会增加这些担忧的因素包括对病人进行门诊随访的障碍以及精神卫生服务系统缺乏能力。

Caring for patients with suicide risk may raise questions and concerns about liability and ethics. In the medical setting, factors that may increase these concerns include barriers to patients following up with outpatient care and a lack of capacity in the mental health service system.

自杀预防共识小组确定了若干策略,以尽量减少对医疗服务提供者或医院的法律诉讼。总的来说,这些策略侧重于遵循国家指导方针,提供以患者为中心的护理,并充分记录每次就诊及决策过程。

The Suicide Prevention Consensus Panel identified several strategies to minimize legal actions against a provider or a hospital. In general, these strategies focus on following national guidelines, providing patient-centered care, and fully documenting each visit and decision-making process.

具体建议包括以下内容:

①提供人性化和以患者为中心的护理,减少对病人的约束,并使用尽可能不受限制的方法来保证患者的安全。

②增加患者选择,尊重患者的自主权。

③获得所有能够提供医疗服务的病人的知情同意。处于危机中或不同意拟议的治疗计划并不等同于没有能力提供知情同意书。

④通过相关人员的证明材料确认患者的病史,并让他们参与治疗和出院计划。

⑤完整记录评估、治疗结果和患者出院的决策支持材料。

Specific recommendations include the following:

①Provide humane and patient-centered care that reduces the need for patient restraint and uses the least restrictive methods possible for keeping patients safe.

②Increase patient choice to demonstrate respect for patients' autonomy.

③ Obtain informed consent for medical treatments from all patients who are able to provide it. Being in a crisis or disagreeing with the proposed treatment plan is not the same as being clinically incompetent.

④ Confirm patients' history with their collaterals and involve them in treatment and discharge planning.

⑤ Fully document evaluations, results, and decisions leading to patient discharge.

附　　录
Appendices

附录1　自杀风险评估量表
Appendix1　Suicide Risk and Assessment Scale

1.1 住院患者自杀危险分层量表

	是（1分）	否（0分）
性别(男)		
年龄(小于20岁或大于45岁)		
抑郁情绪		
曾自杀未遂		
酒精滥用		
丧失理性情绪		
缺乏社会支持		
有周密的自杀计划		
无配偶		
有疾病		

注:该量表总分0~10分,分值越高,表明自杀风险就越高。

0~4分:低风险;5~6分:中度风险;7~10分:高风险。

1.1 Sad Persons

	Yes（1 point）	No（0 point）
Sex(male)		
Age(<20 or >45 years old)		
Depression		
Previous attempt		
Ethanol abuse		
Rational thinking loss		
Social support deficit		
Organized plan		

	Yes（1 point）	No（0 point）
No spouse		
Sickness		

Note：Sad Persons scores range from 0 to 10，where the higher the score，the higher the suicide risk. 0-4：Low risk；5-6：Medium risk；7-10：High risk.

1.2 住院患者心理痛苦温度计

首先，请选择最符合您近一周所经历的平均痛苦水平的数字。

0	1	2	3	4	5	6	7	8	9	10

注：其中0为无痛苦，10为极度痛苦。1~3分为轻度痛苦；4~10分为中重度痛苦，得分越高代表心理痛苦程度越重。

接着，请指出下列哪些选项是引起您痛苦的原因？并在该项目前打"√"。

实际问题：

□没有时间照顾孩子/老人 □没有时间精力做家务 □经济问题

□交通出行 □工作/上学 □周围环境

交往问题：

□与孩子/老人相处 □与伴侣相处 □与亲友相处

□与医护人员相处

情绪问题：

□抑郁 □恐惧 □孤独 □紧张 □悲伤 □担忧

□对日常活动丧失兴趣 □睡眠问题 □记忆力下降/注意力不集中

身体问题：

□外表/形体 □洗澡/穿衣 □呼吸 □排尿改变 □便秘 □腹泻

□进食 □疲乏 □水肿 □发烧 □头晕 □消化不良

□口腔疼痛 □恶心 □鼻子干燥/充血 □疼痛 □性生活

□皮肤干燥 □手/脚麻木 □身体活动受限

信仰/宗教问题：

□信仰/宗教

1.2 Distress Thermometer（DT）

First，choose the number that best matches the average level of pain you've experienced in the last week.

0	1	2	3	4	5	6	7	8	9	10

Note：0 is pain free and 10 is extreme pain. 1~3：mild pain；4~10：moderate to severe pain，and the higher the score，the more severe the psychological pain.

Next，please indicate which of the following options are causing your pain? And tick the item "√".

Practical problems：

☐no time to take care of children/the elderly

☐no time and energy to do housework　　☐financial problems

☐transportation　　☐ work/school　　☐ environment

Communication problems：

☐getting along with children/old people　　☐getting along with partners

☐getting along with relatives and friends　　☐working with medical staff

Emotional problems：

☐depression　☐fear　　☐loneliness　　☐ tension　　☐ sadness　　☐worry

☐loss of interest in daily activities　　☐sleep problems

☐loss of memory/concentration

Physical problems：

☐appearance/form　　☐ bathing/dressing　　☐ breathing

☐changes in urination　☐constipation　　☐ diarrhea　　☐eating

☐fatigue　　☐edema　　☐fever　　☐dizziness　　☐indigestion

☐mouth pain　☐nausea　　☐dry nose/congestion　☐pain　☐sex life

☐dry skin　　☐numbness of hands/feet　　☐limited physical activities

Faith/religion problems：

☐ faith/religion

1.3 患者健康问卷-9

在过去的两周里,你感觉自己被以下症状所困扰的频率是?	完全没有	有过几天	超过一半天数	几乎每天
1.对任何事情都提不起兴趣/感受不到兴趣				
2.感觉沮丧、忧郁或绝望				
3.无法入睡,无法保持睡眠,或睡眠时间过多				
4.感觉乏力或没有精力				
5.没有胃口或过量进食				
6.对自己感到不满(感觉自己是个失败者),或感觉让自己或家人失望				
7.无法集中注意力,比如看报纸或看电视时				
8.行动或说话缓慢,以至于引起旁人注意,或因烦躁而坐立不安				
9.认为死亡或以某种途径伤害自己是解决方式				

注:该量表采用 Likert 4 级评分法,依次计 1~4 分,总分 9~36 分,得分越高,自杀风险越大。

1.3 The Patient Health Questionnaire（PHQ-9）

In the past two weeks, how often have you felt troubled by the following symptoms?	Not at all	Several days	More than half the days	Nearly every day
1. Little interest or pleasure in doing things				
2. Feeling down, depressed, or hopeless				
3. Trouble with falling or staying asleep, or sleeping too much				
4. Feeling tired of having little energy				
5. Poor appetite or overeating				
6. Feeling bad about yourself, or that you are a failure or having let yourself or your family down				
7. Trouble with concentrating on things, such as reading the newspaper or watching television				
8. Moving or speaking so slowly that others could have noticed, or the opposite, being so fidgety or restless that you have been moving a lot more than usual				

In the past two weeks, how often have you felt troubled by the following symptoms?	Not at all	Several days	More than half the days	Nearly every day
9. Thoughts that you would be better off dead, or of hurting yourself in some way				

Note: The scale adopts the Likert Level 4 scoring method, which counts 1 to 4 points in turn, with a total score of 9 to 36 points. The higher the score, the greater the risk of suicide.

1.4 患者安全筛查问卷

	是	否	不确定
1.在过去2周内,您是否情绪低落、抑郁或绝望?			
2.在过去2周内,您是否有过自杀的想法?			
3.您是否有过自杀行为,是什么时候发生的?			

注:选项为"是""否""不确定",若患者近2周内有自杀意念或近6个月内有自杀行为,则被认为存在自杀风险。

1.4 Patient Safety Screener（PSS）

	Yes	No	Uncertain
1.Have you been depressed, grieved or hopeless in the past 2 weeks?			
2.Have you had suicide thoughts in the past 2 weeks?			
3.Have you ever suicided and when did it happen?			

Note: The options are "Yes", "no" or "uncertain". If the patient had suicide ideation in the last 2 weeks or suicide behavior in the last 6 months, the patient was considered to be at risk of suicide.

1.5 自杀可能性量表

	从来没有	偶尔	大部分时间	几乎每天
1.当我发狂时,我扔东西				
2.我感到很多人深切的关心着我				
3.我觉得自己常常很冲动				
4.我认为事情糟糕得无法与人分享				
5.我觉得自己肩负着太多责任				
6.我觉得有很多我能做也值得我去做的事情				
7.为了惩罚他人,我考虑过自杀				
8.我对他人怀有敌意				

	从来没有	偶尔	大部分时间	几乎每天
9.我感到与人们疏离				
10.我觉得人们欣赏真实的我				
11.我觉得如果我死了,很多人会感到难过				
12.我感觉很孤独,无法忍受				
13.别人对我怀有敌意				
14.我觉得如果一切可以重来,我将会对我的生活做出很多改变				
15.我觉得我有很多事情做不好				
16.我在寻找并坚持我喜欢的工作方面有困难				
17.我觉得当我离去的时候,没有人会想念我				
18.对我来说,事情都在向好的方向发展				
19.我觉得人们对我的期望太高				
20.我觉得我需要为自己曾经想过和做过的事情而惩罚自己				
21.我觉得这世界不值得我再继续生活下去了				
22.我很认真地规划未来				
23.我觉得我没有太多可以依赖的朋友				
24.我觉得如果我死了别人会过得更好				
25.我觉得死亡会减轻痛苦				
26.我觉得/曾觉得和母亲关系很亲近				
27.我觉得/曾觉得和朋友关系很亲近				
28.我对事情向好的方向发展不抱期望				
29.我觉得人们不赞同我或我所做的事情				
30.我曾经想过怎样自杀				
31.我有经济压力				
32.我想自杀				
33.我感觉疲惫,无精打采				
34.当我发狂时,我毁坏东西				
35.我觉得/曾觉得和父亲关系很亲近				
36.我觉得无论在哪我都无法高兴				

注:该量表采用 Likert 4 级评分法,依次计 1~4 分,总分 36~144 分,得分越高,自杀风险越大。

1.5 Suicide Probability Scale（SPS）

	Not at all	Once in a while	Most of the time	Nearly every day
1. When I'm mad, I throw things				
2. I feel that many people care deeply about me				
3. I think I'm often impulsive				
4. I think things are too bad to share				
5. I feel I have too much responsibility on my shoulders				
6. I think there are a lot of things I can do and are worth doing				
7. To punish others, I considered suicide				
8. I feel hostility towards others				
9. I feel alienated from people				
10. I think people appreciate me for who I am				
11. I think if I die, a lot of people would feel sad				
12. I feel so lonely that I can not bear it				
13. I am treated with hostility				
14. I feel that if I could do it all over again, I would make a lot of changes in my life				
15. I think there are a lot of things I can't do well				
16. I have trouble finding and sticking to a job I like				
17. I don't think anyone would miss me when I'm gone				
18. For me, things are getting better				
19. I think people expect too much of me				
20. I feel I need to punish myself for what I have thought and done				
21. I don't think the world is worth living in anymore				
22. I planed my future very carefully				
23. I don't think I have many friends to rely on				
24. I think people would be better off if I die				
25. I think death would ease the pain				
26. I feel very close to my mother				
27. I feel very close to my friends				
28. I don't expect things to turn out well				
29. I feel like people don't agree with me or what I'm doing				

	Not at all	Once in a while	Most of the time	Nearly every day
30. I ever thought about how to kill myself				
31. I'm under financial pressure				
32. I want to commit suicide				
33. I feel tired and listless				
34. When I go crazy, I destroy things				
35. I feel very close to my father				
36. I don't think I can be happy anywhere				

Note: The scale adopts the Likert Level 4 scoring method, which counts 1 to 4 points in turn, with a total score of 36 to 144 points. The higher the score, the greater the risk of suicide.

1.6 住院患者自杀风险评估量表

在过去一个月内,患者是否有以下问题的困扰?请在相应的栏目里打钩(√)	是（1分）	否（0分）
1.患者患有难以治愈的严重躯体疾病(如恶性肿瘤、重要器官衰竭等)		
2.患者发生了影响躯体某部位功能的并发症(如毁容、畸形等)		
3.患者经常感到身体疼痛难忍(疼痛是由疾病引起的)		
4.患者失眠(失眠是由疾病引起)		
5.患者经常觉得事情不可能好转,对未来悲观失望		
6.患者采取消极(如逃避、自责)的应对方式来应对困难和挫折		
7.患者对自我的评价(即自己对自己的看法、想法)是消极悲观的		
8.患者经常情绪低落,感到抑郁		
9.患者有精神方面相关症状(如精神分裂症、焦虑症、边缘型人格障碍等)		
10.患者经常表现得很冲动(即因微小刺激突然爆发出冲动性或攻击性行为)		
11.患者对任何事情都追求尽善尽美(即完美主义)		
12.患者曾经采取过伤害自己的行为		
13.患者说过不想活了,觉得生活没有意义等话语		
14.患者生活习惯发生了改变(如开始大量饮酒、使用药物助眠等)		
15.患者发生了严重的家庭矛盾		
16.患者家人或朋友曾经采取过伤害自己的行为		
17.患者遭受了重大挫折		
18.患者人际关系处于紧张状态		

注:条目"是"为1分,"否"为0分,总分0~18分。当分值≥8分时,可判定为患者有自杀风险。

1.6 Inpatient Suicide Risk Assessment Scale （I-SRAS）

In the past month，did the patient have any of the following problems？ Please tick the appropriate box.	Yes （1 point）	No （0 point）
1. The patient suffered from a serious physical disease that was difficult to cure（e.g., malignant tumor，failure of vital organs，etc.）		
2. The patient developed complications（disfigurement，deformity，etc.）that affected the function of certain parts of the body		
3. The patient often experienced physical pain（pain caused by illness）		
4. The patient suffered from insomnia（insomnia caused by disease）		
5. The patient often felt that things couldn't get better and was pessimistic about the future		
6. The patient coped with difficulties and setbacks by adopting negative coping styles such as avoidance and self-blame		
7. The patient had a negative and pessimistic view of himself/herself		
8. The patient often felt low and depressed		
9. The patient had psychotic symptoms（schizophrenia，anxiety，borderline personality disorder，etc.）		
10. The patient was often impulsive（i.e.，sudden bursts of impulsive or aggressive behavior due to a small stimulus）		
11. The patient strived for perfection in everything（i.e.，perfectionism）		
12. The patient has taken actions that hurt him/her		
13. The patient has said that he/she did not want to live，feeling life had no meaning and other words		
14. There were changes in the patient's lifestyle（e.g.，starting to drink a lot of alcohol，using drugs to help sleep，etc.）		
15. The patient had a serious family conflict		
16. His/Her Family members or friends have taken actions that hurt him/her		
17. The patient suffered a major setback		
18. The patient's interpersonal relationship was in a state of tension		

Note："Yes" is 1 point，"No" is 0 points，and the total score is 0 to 18 points.

When the score≥8 points，it can be determined that the patient is at risk of suicide.

1.7 广泛性焦虑障碍量表

	完全不会	好几天	超过一周	几乎每天
1.感觉紧张、焦虑或急切				
2.不能停止或控制担忧				
3.对各种各样的事情担忧过多				
4.很难放松下来				
5.由于不安而无法静坐				
6.变得容易烦恼或急躁				
7.感到似乎将有可怕的事情发生而害怕				

注释：每个条目0~3分，总分0~21分。

0~4：正常；5~9：轻度风险；10~14：中度风险；15~21：重度风险。

1.7 Generalized Anxiety Disorder Scale（GAD-7）

	Not at all	Several days	More than a week	Almost every day
1. To feel nervous, or anxious				
2. Can't stop or control worry				
3. To worry too much about all kinds of things				
4. Hard to relax				
5. Unable to sit still because of uneasiness				
6. To become easily annoyed or irritable				
7. To feel as if something terrible is going to happen and being afraid				

Note: Each item is 0-3 points, with a total score of 0-21 points.

0~4：normal；5~9: mild risk；10~14: moderate risk；15~21：severe risk.

附录 2　分享患者健康信息
Appendix 2　Sharing Patient Health Information

健康保险流通与责任法案允许卫生保健提供者共享信息的情形如下：

1. 与参与患者护理过程的家庭成员、朋友或其他人沟通时。

2. 与成年人患者的家属沟通时。

3. 当患者是未成年，与未成年人患者的监护人沟通时。

4. 考虑患者同意或反对共享他们信息的能力。

5. 当患者药物治疗或其他治疗失败时，应告知患者的家庭成员、朋友或其他人。

6. 倾听家属讲述他们所爱的人接受心理健康治疗的情况。

7. 当患者对自己或他人造成严重或迫在眉睫的伤害时，与家人、执法人员或其他人进行沟通。

8. 与执法部门沟通释放一名急诊精神病院的病人时。

HIPPA permits health care providers to：

1. Communicate with a patient's family members, friends, or others involved in the patient's care.

2. Communicate with his/her family members when the patient is an adult.

3. Communicate with the parent of a patient who is a minor.

4. Consider the patient's capacity to agree or object to the sharing of their information.

5. Involve a patient's family members, friends, or others in dealing with patient failures to adhere to medication or other therapy.

6. Listen to the family members about their loved ones receiving mental health treatment.

7. Communicate with his/her family members, law enforcement, or others when the patient presents a serious and imminent threat of harm to self or others.

8. Communicate to law enforcement about the release of a patient brought in for an emergency psychiatric hold.

附录3　关怀性联系样本资料
Appendix3　Caring Contacts Sample Materials

关怀性联系是基于证据的干预措施。对于希望实施这种干预的医院，下面提供了一些相关护理资料的样本。这些样本是基于美国各地危机中心、医院和退伍军人事务部医护人员的自杀预防专家和研究人员的工作。它们可以适用于您的急诊科和当前的技术选项（如短信、电子邮件）。

Caring contacts is an evidence-based intervention. For hospitals wishing to implement this intervention, a few samples of caring contact materials are provided below. These samples are based on the work of suicide prevention professionals and researchers using caring contacts in crisis centers, hospitals, and VA settings across the Unites States. They can be adapted for use in your ED and for current technology options(e.g., text messaging, e-mail).

样函1

尊敬的***：

你离开大学医院已经有一段时间了，我们希望你一切顺利。如果你想给我们寄一张便条，我们很乐意收到你的来信。

最美好的祝愿，Smith 医生

Sample 1.

Dear <<First Name>>

It has been a little while since you were at University Hospital, and we hope things are going well for you. If you would like to send us a note we would enjoy hearing from you.

Best wishes, Dr. Smith

样函2

尊敬的***：

很高兴在大学医院见到你。我们希望你一切都好。我们记得你说你享受做祖父（母）。我们希望你今年春天有时间和你的孙子一起度过。我们只是想给你发个短讯，让你知道我们挂念着你并且希望你一切顺利。如果您愿意给我们回信并给我们发一份您最新的情况，我们将很高兴收到您的来信。

此致

Sandra Lamont, LCSW

Sample 2.

Dear <<First Name>>

It was great to meet you at University Hospital. We hope you are doing well. We remember that you said you enjoyed being a grandparent. We hope you're getting time to spend with your grandchildren this spring. We just want to send a quick note to let you know we are thinking about you and wish you well. If you'd like to reply to us and send us an update, we would be happy to hear from you.

Sincerely,

Sandra Lamont, LCSW

样函3:俄克拉荷马城退伍军人医疗中心

该项目每季度向有自杀风险的患者发送有关健康和心理健康信息的新闻通讯。案例管理员基于此目的提供的随访信函空白处手写了这一关怀短信。

你好,***先生/女士,

我希望自我们上次谈话以来你一直做得很好。如果有什么我能帮忙的,请打电话给我。

Bryan Stice 博士
自杀预防案例主任
(电话:**********)

Sample 3. Oklahoma City VA Medical Center

This program sends quarterly newsletters to patients at risk of suicide with information about health and mental health. The caring note is hand-written by the case manager in a space in the newsletter provided for this purpose.

Hi <<Mr. or Ms.>> <<Last Name>>,

I hope you have been doing well since we last spoke. Give me a call if there's anything I can do for you.

Bryan Stice, PhD
Suicide Prevention Case Manager
<<Phone>>

参考文献

References

［1］ 崔黎黎,孙婷婷,董光辉.当代中国自杀及自杀行为流行病学特征及干预［J］.医学综述,2009,15(23):3655-3658.

［2］ 邓云龙,钟瑜,潘辰.躯体疾病住院患者自杀意念预警量表初步编制［J］.中华行为医学与脑科学杂志,2014,23(5):469-471.

［3］ 胡德英,柳丽茗,邓先锋,等.568例急诊科自杀未遂患者特征分析与管理对策［J］.护理学杂志,2018,33(18):15-17.

［4］ 丁小萍,胡德英,万青,等.湖北省45所综合医院非精神科住院患者自杀行为的调查［J］.中华护理杂志,2019,54(6):861-866.

［5］ 毛世清,胡德英,向莉,陈莹.急诊科服毒自杀患者医疗费用影响因素分析［J］.中国病案,2020,21(3):71-74.

［6］ 孟艳君,王斌全,朱瑞芳,等.综合医院住院病人人格障碍、抑郁、焦虑与自杀意念的相关性［J］.护理研究,2020,34(11):1898-1904.

［7］ 徐东,张学立,曹孔敬,许永臣,费立鹏.农村地区农药与非农药自杀医疗费用负担分析［J］.中国心理卫生杂志,2008(4):308.

［8］ American Psychiatric Association. Practice guideline for the assessment and treatment of patients with suicidal behaviors［J］. The American Journal of Psychiatry,2003,160(11):1-60.

［9］ Ang L. Reducing inpatient suicide rates: the success of a suicide management programme in a general hospital［J］. General Hospital Psychiatry,2018(54): 60-61.

［10］ Ashmore R, Hemingway S, Lees J, et al.Mental health nursing: assessing therapeutic intervention used by NHS direct nurse advisers［J］. British Journal of Nursing, 2001,10(10):662-664.

［11］ Austin W. Psychiatric & mental nursing for Canadian practice［M］. Philadelphia: Lippincott Williams & Wilkins,2008.

［12］ Bachmann S. Epidemiology of suicide and the psychiatric perspective［J］.International Journal of Environmental Research and Public Health, 2018, 15(7):1425.

[13] Ball B , White J. Wondering and wanderings: ongoing conversations about suicide prevention[J]. Visions: BC's Mental Health and Addictions Journal, 2005,2(7): 4-5.

[14] Barling J, Brown R. Credentials and education needs for contemporary mental health nurses[J]. International Journal of Psychiatric Nursing Research, 2001(6):726-736.

[15] Barlow C, Morrison H. Survivors of suicide: emerging counseling strategies [J]. Journal of Psychosocial Nursing and Mental Health Services, 2002, 40(1): 28-39.

[16] Bennett S, Daly J, Kirkwood J, et al. Establishing evidence-based standards of practice for suicidal patients in emergency medicine[J]. Topics in Emergency Medicine, 2006,28(2):138-143.

[17] Berlim M T, Mattevi B S, Pavanello D P , et al. Psychache and suicidality in adult mood disordered outpatients in Brazil[J]. Suicide & Life-Threatening Behavior, 2003,33(3):242-248.

[18] Browne A J, Varcoe C. Critical cultural perspectives and health care involving Aboriginal peoples[J]. Contemporary Nurse,2006, 22(2): 155-167.

[19] Brugha T , Rampes H, Jenkins R. Surely you take complementary and alternative medicine? [J].Psychiatric Bulletin,2004(28): 36-39.

[20] Burgess A W. Advanced practice psychiatric nursing[M]. Stamford, CT: Appletone & Lange, 1998.

[21] Canner J K, Giuliano K, Selvarajah S, et al. Emergency department visits for attempted suicide and self harm in the USA: 2006-2013[J]. Epidemiology and Psychiatric Sciences,2018, 27(1) : 94-102.

[22] Captain C. Is your patient a suicide risk? [J].Nursing, 2006(36):43-47.

[23] Carlen P, Bengtsson A. Suicidal patients as experienced by psychiatric nurses in inpatient care[J]. International Journal of Mental Health Nursing, 2007(16): 257-265.

[24] Cavoukian A.A guide to the personal health information protection act[M]. Toronto: Information and Privacy Commissioner of Ontario,2004.

[25] Cedereke M , Ojehagen A. Patients'needs during the year after a suicide attempt. A secondary analysis of a randomised controlled intervention study[J].Social Psychiatry & Psychiatric Epidemiology,2002, 37(8): 357-363.

[26] Crawford M J, Turnbull G , Wessely S. Deliberate self harm assessment by accident and emergency staff an intervention study[J]. Journal of Accident

and Emergency Medicine,1998, 15(1):18-22.

[27] Cutcliffe J R, Barker P. Considering the care of the suicidal client and the case for 'engagement and inspiring hope' or 'observations' [J]. Journal of Psychiatric and Mental Health Nursing, 2002(9):611-621.

[28] Cutcliffe J R, Barker P. The nurses' Global Assessment of Suicide Risk (NGASR): developing a tool for clinical practice[J]. Journal of Psychiatric and Mental Health Nursing, 2004(11):393-400.

[29] Dafoe B, Monk L. Suicide postvention is prevention: A proactive planning workbook for communities affected by youth suicide[J]. Visions: BC's Mental Health and Addictions Journal,2005, 2(7): 34-35.

[30] Diaconu G, Turecki G. Panic disorder and suicidality: is comorbidity with depression the key? [J].Journal of Affective Disorder, 2007,104(1): 203-209.

[31] Dlugacz Y D, Restifo A, Scanlon K, et al. Safety strategies to prevent suicide in multiple health care environments[J]. Joint Commission Journal on Quality and Safety,2003, 29(6), 267-278.

[32] Eagles J M, Carson D P, Begg A, et al.Suicide prevention: a study of patients' views[J]. The British Journal of Psychiatry,2003(182): 261-265.

[33] Ernst E, Rand J I, Stevinson C. Complementary therapies for depression: an overview[J]. Archives General Psychiatry, 1998,55(11):1026-1032.

[34] Farrow T L. Owning their expertise: Why nurses use "no suicide" contracts rather than their own assessments[J]. International Journal of Mental Health Nursing, 2002,11(4): 214-219.

[35] Farrow T L."No suicide contracts" in community crisis situations: a conceptual analysis[J]. Journal of Psychiatric & Mental Health Nursing, 2003, 10(2):199-202.

[36] Gaynes B N, West S L, Ford C A, et al. Screening for suicide risk in adults: a summary of the evidence for the U.S. Preventive Services Task Force[J]. Annals of Internal Medicine, 2004,140(10): 822-835.

[37] Gough K. Guidelines for managing self-harm in a forensic setting[J]. British Journal of Forensic Practice,2005, 7(2): 10-14.

[38] Graham I D, Harrison M B, Brouwers M, et al. Facilitating the use of evidence in practice: evaluating and adapting clinical practice guidelines for local use by health care organizations[J]. Journal of Obstetric, Gynecologic, and Neonatal Nursing, 2002,31(5): 599-611.

[39] Holkup P A. Evidence-based protocol: elderly suicide-secondary prevention [M]. Iowa City, IA: University of Iowa Gerontological Nursing, 2003

[40] Horrocks J, House A, Owens D. Establishing a clinical database for hospital attendances because of self-harm [J]. Psychiatric Bulletin, 2004 (28): 137-139.

[41] Jones J, Ward M, Wellman N, et al. Psychiatric inpatients' experience of nursing observation. A United Kingdom perspective[J]. Journal of Psychosocial Nursing & Mental Health Services, 2000,38(12): 10-20.

[42] Javdani S, Sadeh N, Verona E. Suicidality as a function of impulsivity, callous - unemotional traits, and depressive symptoms in youth[J]. Journal of Abnormal Psychology,2011,120(2): 400-413.

[43] Keilp J G, Sackeim H A, et al. Neuropsychological dysfunction in depressed suicide attempters[J]. The American Journal of Psychiatry,2001, 158 (5): 735-741.

[44] Klonsky E D, May A M. The Three-Step Theory (3ST): A new theory of suicide rooted in the "ideation-to-action" framework[J]. International Journal of Cognitive Therapy,2015,8(2):114-129.

[45] Kroll J. No-suicide contracts as a suicide prevention strategy[J]. Psychiatric Times, 2007,24(8):60.

[46] Kleiman E M. Riskind J H, et al. The moderating role of social support on the Rrelationship between impulsivity and suicide risk[J]. Crisis: The Journal of Crisis Intervention and Suicide Prevention,2012,33 (5): 273-279.

[47] LeGris J, van Reekum R. The neuropsychological correlates of borderline personality disorder and suicidal behaviour[J]. The Canadian Journal of Psychiatry,2016, 51 (3): 131-142.

[48] Linehan M M. Cognitive-behavioral treatment of borderline personality disorder[M]. New York: Guildford Press,1993.

[49] MacLeod A K, Tata P, Kentish J, et al. Anxiety, depression, and explanation-based pessimism for future positive and negative events[J]. Clinical Psychology & Psychotherapy, 1997,4(1):15-24.

[50] Mamo D C. Managing suicidality in schizophrenia[J]. Canadian Journal of Psychiatry, 2007,52(6):59.

[51] Mann J J, Apter A, Bertolote J, et al. Suicide prevention strategies: a systematic review[J]. Journal of the American Medical Association,2005,

294(16): 2064-2074.

[52] Maslow A H. A theory of human motivation[J]. Psychological Review, 1943 (50):370-396.

[53] McMain S. Effectiveness of psychosocial treatments on suicidality in personality disorders[J]. Canadian Journal of Psychiatry, 2007,52(6): 103-114.

[54] National Collaborating Centre for Mental Health. Self-harm: the short-term physical and psychological management and secondary prevention of self-harm in primary and secondary care[M]. London, UK: National Institute for Clinical Excellence,2004.

[55] New Zealand Guidelines Group (NZGG) and Ministry of Health. The assessment and management of people at risk of suicide[M/OL]. (2003-05-01)[2021-01-20]. https://www.health.govt.nz/publication/assessment-and-management-people-risk-suicide.

[56] O'Brien L, Cole R. Close-observation areas in acute psychiatric units: a literature review[J]. International Journal of Mental Health Nursing, 2003, 12(3): 165-176.

[57] Ostman M, Kjellin L. Stigma by association: psychological factors in relatives of people with mental illness[J]. British Journal of Psychiatry, 2002(181): 494-498.

[58] Pirkis J, Burgess P, Meadows G, et al. Self-reported needs for care among persons who have suicidal ideation or who have attempted suicide[J]. Psychiatric Services, 2001,52(3): 381-383.

[59] Proctor N G. Parasuicide, self-harm and suicide in Aboriginal people in rural Australia: a review of the literature with implications for mental health nursing practice[J]. International Journal of Nursing Practice, 2005, 11(5): 237-241.

[60] Ramsden I. Cultural safety in nursing education in Aotearoa (New Zealand) [J]. Nursing Praxis in New Zealand, 1993,8(3):4-10.

[61] Ramsden, I. Cultural safety/Kawa whakaruruhau ten years on: a personal overview[J]. Nursing Praxis in New Zealand, 2000,15(1):4-12.

[62] Reynolds T, O'Shaughnessy M, Walker L, et al. Safe and supportive observation in practice: a clinical governance project[J]. Mental Health Practice, 2005,8(8):13-16.

[63] Royal College of Psychiatrists (RCP). Assessment following self-harm in adults[M/OL]. (2003-05-01)[2021-01-20]. https://www.researchgate.net/

publication/241885806_Assessment_of_Deliberate_Self-harm_in_Adults.

[64] Royal College of Psychiatrists (RCP). Better services for people who self-harm: quality standards for healthcare professionals [M/OL]. (2003-05-01) [2021-01-20]. http://www.rcpsych.ac.uk/auditselfharm.htm, 2006.

[65] Rudd M D, Mandrusiak M, Joiner T E. The case against no‑suicide contracts: the commitment to treatment statement as a practice alternative [J]. Journal of Clinical Psychology, 2006, 62(2): 243-251.

[66] Smith A R. Witte T K, et al. Revisiting impulsivity in suicide: implications for civil liability of third parties[J]. Behavioral Sciences & the Law, 2008, 26(6): 779-797.

[67] Sakinofsky I. The aftermath of suicide: managing survivors' bereavement [J]. The Canadian Journal of Psychiatry, 2007, 52(6): 129-136.

[68] Sakinsofsky I. The current evidence base for the clinical care of suicidal patients: strengths and weaknesses[J]. The Canadian Journal of Psychiatry, 2007: 52(6): 7-20.

[69] Sakinofsky I. Treating suicidality in depressive illness. Part 2: does treatment cure or cause suicidality? [J]. The Canadian Journal of Psychiatry, 2007, 52(6): 35-45.

[70] Sher L, Oquendo M A, Mann J J. Risk of suicide in mood disorders [J]. Clinical Neuroscience Research, 2001, 1(5): 337-344.

[71] Simon R I. Assessing and managing suicide risk: guidelines for clinically based risk management[J]. Washington: American Psychiatric Publishing, 2008.

[72] Sullivan A M, Barron C T, Bezmen J, et al. The safe treatment of the suicidal patient in an adult inpatient setting: a proactive preventive approach [J]. Psychiatric Quarterly, 2005, 76(1): 67-83.

[73] Taylor C. Clinical problem‑solving in nursing: insights from the literature [J]. Journal of Advanced Nursing, 2000, 31(4): 842-849.

[74] Van Orden K A, Witte T K, et al. The interpersonal theory of suicide[J]. Psychological Review, 2010, 117(2): 575-600.

[75] Waldram J B. The way of the pipe: aboriginal spirituality and symbolic healing in Canadian prisons[M]. Peterborough, ON: Broadview Press, 1997.

[76] Weier K M, Beal M W. Complementary therapies as adjuncts in the treatment of postpartum depression [J]. Journal of Midwifery & Women's Health, 2004, 49(2): 96-104.

[77] Wiklander M, Samuelsson M, Asberg M. Shame reactions after suicide attempt[J]. Scandinavian Journal of Caring Sciences, 2003,17(3):293-300.

[78] Williams J W, Mulrow C D, Chiquette E, et al. A systematic review of newer pharmacotherapies for depression in adults: evidence report summary [J]. Annals of Internal Medicine,2000, 132(9):743-756.

[79] Wilson A, Clark S. South Australian suicide postvention project report to mental health services, department of health[M]. Adelaide: Department of General Practice,2005.

[80] Yeager K R, Saveanu R, Roberts A R, et al. Measured response to identified suicide risk and violence: what you need to know about psychiatric patient safety[J]. Brief Treatment and Crisis Intervention,2005(5):121-141.

[81] Yurgelun-Todd D A, Bueler C E, McGlade E C,et al. Neuroimaging correlates of traumatic brain injury and suicidal behavior [J]. Journal of Head Trauma Rehabilitation ,2011,26 (4): 276-289.

中英文名词对照索引

Chinese and English Noun Comparison Index

A

自杀未遂 attempted suicide
利他型自杀 altruistic suicide
失范型自杀 anomic suicide
替代疗法 alternative therapy
焦虑 anxiety
美国精神病学会 American psychiatric association，APA
攻击性 aggression

B

边缘型人格障碍 borderline personality disorder
简要患者教育 brief patient education

C

哥伦比亚自杀评估分类法 Columbia Classification Algorithm of Suicide Assessment ，C-SACA
自杀死亡 committed suicide
文化安全 cultural safety
认知行为疗法 Cognitive Behavioral Therapy，CBT
慢性疼痛 chronic pain
慢性压力源 chronic stressor
护理决策 care decision
反移情 countertransference
关怀联络 caring contact
危机热线 crisis hotline

D

个性化护理决策 decision-making for individualized client care
震颤性谵妄 delirium tremens

辩证行为疗法 Dialectical Behavioral Therapy，DBT
抑郁 depression
决策支持工具 decision support tool
出院计划清单 discharge planning checklist
文书记录 documentation
心理痛苦温度计 Distress Thermometer，DT

E

基于证据的护理实践 evidence-based nursing practice
电休克疗法 Electro-Convulsive Therapy，ECT
利己型自杀 egoistic suicide

F

焦点团体访谈 focus group interview
随访 follow-up
宿命型自杀 fatalistic suicide

G

整体功能评定量表 Global Assessment of Functioning ，GAF

H

健康中国 Healthy Chinese
住院患者 hospitalized patient
绝望 hopelessness

I

国际疾病分类法 International Classification of Diseases，ICD
跨学科团队 interdisciplinary team
指示性筛查 indicated screening
失眠 insomnia
冲动 impulsiveness
住院患者自杀风险评估量表 Inpatient Suicide Risk Assessment Scale，ISRAS

L

致命自杀方式的限制 lethal means counseling

习得的自杀能力 learned suicidal ability

M

多部门自杀预防策略 multisectoral suicide prevention strategy

马斯洛层次理论 maslow's hierarchy of needs

改良电休克疗法 Modified Electro Convulsive Therapy，MECT

精神疾病 mental disorder

多轴诊断 multi-axis diagnosis

调动资源 mobilizing resources

多学科治疗团队 multidisciplinary team，MDT

激励性谈话技巧 motivational conversation technique

N

不自杀合同 no-suicide contract

P

心理解剖 psycho-anatomy，PA

累赘感知 perceived burdensomeness

同伴讨论 peer debriefing

酒精性癫痫发作 potential alcohol-related seizure

心理疗法 psychotherapy

精神药理学 psychopharmacology

创伤后应激障碍 Post-Traumatic Stress Disorder，PTSD

保护因素 protective factor

初级筛查 primary screening

初级筛查工具 primary screening tool

患者披露 patient disclosure

障碍因素 potential barrier

初级保健提供者 Primary Care Provider，PCP

患者健康问卷-9 Patient Health Questionnaire-9，PHQ-9

患者安全筛查问卷 Patient Safety Screener，PSS

R

根本原因分析 root cause analysis

风险评估 risk assessment

危险因素 risk factor

快速转介 rapid referral

风险管理 risk management

减轻责任担忧 reducing liability concerns

S

自杀守门人 suicide gatekeeper

自杀意念 suicide ideation

自杀准备 suicide preparation

自杀计划 suicide plan

应激—易感理论 stress-susceptibility theory

自杀人际理论 suicide interpersonal theory

自杀扭力理论 strain theory of suicide

耻辱感 stigma

安全的物理环境 safe physical environment

精神分裂症 schizophrenia

睡眠障碍 sleep disorder

物质戒断 substance withdrawal

同性取向 same-sex orientation

性创伤 sexual trauma

二级筛查 secondary screening

选择性筛查 selective screening

安全计划 safety plan

美国自杀预防资源中心 Suicide Prevention Resource Centre，SPRC

自杀预防合同 suicide prevention contract

社会支持网络 social support network

自杀风险评估量表 Sad Persons

自杀可能性量表 Suicide Probability Scale，SPS

T

归属受挫 thwarted belongingness

自杀三阶段理论 three-stage theory of suicide

创伤性脑损伤 Traumatic Brain Injury，TBI

治疗关系 therapeutic relationship

创伤性生活事件 traumatic life event

移情 transference

治疗环境 treatment setting

U

普遍筛查 universal screening

V

替代性创伤 vicarious traumatization
小品文 vignette

W

世界卫生组织 World Health Organization，WHO
预警信号 warning sign

自杀是一个严重的公共卫生问题。据世界卫生组织（WHO）统计，每年有近80万人自杀，至少200万人自杀未遂，自杀是15—29岁人群的第二大死因。中国的自杀人数约占全球自杀人数的10％。

Suicide is a serious public health problem. According to statistics from the World Health Organization（WHO），nearly 800,000 people commit suicide each year，and at least 2 million people attempt suicide. Suicide is the second leading cause of death among people aged 15—29. The number of suicides in China accounts for about 10％ of the global suicides.

在我国，住院患者自杀率是普通人群的4—5倍。自杀反映了社会各发展阶段经济、卫生、教育等方面问题，不仅危及患者生命，给家庭带来巨大精神痛苦，甚至威胁社会的和谐与稳定。健康中国背景下，医护人员面临着严峻的挑战。

In China，the suicide rate of hospitalized patients is 4 to 5 times that of the general population. Suicide reflects the economic，health，education and other aspects of social development stages. It endangers the lives of patients，brings huge mental pain to their families，and even threatens the harmony and stability of society. In the context of healthy Chinese，medical staff are in the face of serious challenges.

当代著名作家余华先生在《活着》一书中说过："人只要活着，就有希望。人只要活着就是一种胜利。生不可选，死不该选。"自杀是可以通过及时的、基于证据的、低成本的干预措施来预防的。为了使国家应对措施有效，需要一项全面的多部门自杀预防战略。

The famous contemporary writer Mr. Yu Hua said in his book *Living*："As long as people live，there is hope. As long as people live，there is a victory. There is no choice for life，no choice for death." Suicide can be prevented through timely，evidence-based，low-cost interventions. For national response measures to be effective，a comprehensive multisectoral suicide prevention strategy is needed.

住院患者自杀是威胁患者安全的重大事件。护理人员在住院期间与患者接触最多，在预防患者自杀、保障患者安全方面具有不可替代的作用。培训护理人员成为自杀守门人，识别具有自杀倾向的患者，减少住院患者自杀事件的发生，具有重要的现实意义。国内一些学者围绕住院患者自杀预防开展了一些探索，但内容较分散，缺乏系统性和全面性。

Suicide of inpatients is a major event threatening the safety of patients. Nursing staff have the most contact with the patients during their hospitalization, and they play an irreplaceable role in preventing suicide and ensuring the patients'safety. It is of great practical significance to train nursing staff to become suicide gatekeepers, identify the patients with suicide tendency, and reduce the occurrence of suicides among inpatients. Some domestic scholars have carried out some explorations around suicide prevention of hospitalized patients, but the content is scattered and lacks systematicity and comprehensiveness.

本书作者胡德英主任护师从事护理工作三十余年，深入研究住院患者自杀近十年。她带领的团队在研究前期运用焦点团体访谈、根本原因分析法、5M1E 法、心理解剖法、问卷调查法等定性与定量相结合的方法，深入研究住院患者自杀风险因素，创新了"住院患者自杀原因剖析—护士分层培训—自杀风险筛查与评估—自杀预防与干预"等一系列患者自杀风险管理模式。

Hu Deying, professor of nursing, one of the authors of this book, has been engaged in nursing for more than 30 years, and has been studying inpatient suicide for nearly ten years. In the early stage of the study, her team adopted focus group interviews, root cause analysis, 5M1E, psycho-anatomy, questionnaires, and other qualitative and quantitative methods to deeply study the risk factors of suicide in hospitalized patients. A series of management models for risk of suicide have been innovated such as "Analysis of the reasons of suicide in inpatients—Stratified training of nurses —Screening and assessment of suicide risk—Interventions and preventions of suicide".

研究团队率先对经历患者自杀的护士进行针对性的心理干预，医护人员不再避讳公开谈论自杀话题，这打破了"禁区"，在全院形成了良好的预防患者自杀安全文化氛围，住院患者自杀行为发生率呈下降趋势。前期的研究为撰写本书提供了科学的理论指导，也为临床实践打下了坚实的基础。

The research team took the lead in targeted psychological intervention for nurses who have experienced suicide attempts by patients , and medical staff are no longer afraid of talking about suicide, breaking the "forbidden zone", forming a good culture of suicide prevention safety in the hospital, and the incidence of suicide behavior in hospitalized patients shows a downward trend. The previous research provided scientific theoretical guidance for writing this book, and laid a solid foundation for clinical practice.

本书在国家自然科学基金面上项目"安全文化视角下住院患者自杀风险评估指标体系及危机管理模型构建"(NO.71673100)资助支持下出版。研究团队参考国外患者自杀风险管理相关共识指南,结合临床实践经验,编制了这本《患者自杀风险管理手册》。本书为我国患者自杀风险评估与预防干预工作提供有力的实践指导,帮助临床管理者、医务人员、自杀患者及家属应对自杀问题。

This book is published under the support of the National Natural Science Foundation of China , a general project of "Establishment of Suicide Risk Assessment Index System and Crisis Management Model for Inpatients under the Perspective of Safety Culture" (NO.71673100). The research team referred to overseas consensus and guidelines related to suicide risk management for patients, combining with experience of clinical nursing practice, and compiled this *Handbook of Patient Suicide Risk Management*. This book provides powerful practical guidance for suicide risk assessment and prevention and intervention of patients in our country, and helps clinical managers, medical staff, suicide patients and their families cope with suicide.

全书由自杀风险患者护理概述、患者自杀风险评估、患者自杀预防干预、自杀风险患者的随访、自杀风险患者的文书记录五个部分组成。通过汉英对照,力求照顾到各级各类医院读者的阅读需求,拓展读者的知识面。此外,书中插入了一些实践框与小品文等,结合相关自杀典型案例,提高读者的阅读兴趣,帮助读者更广泛、深入地理解和把握自杀预防实践要求,能够更好地将理论与实践相结合。

The book is composed of five parts: summary of nursing care for patients at risk of suicide, assessment of patients at risk of suicide, preventions and interventions in patients with suicide, follow-up for patients at risk of suicide, and documentation of patients at risk of suicide. Through the comparison in Chinese and English, we strive to cater for the reading needs of readers of different levels and ages, and expand readers' knowledge. In addition, some practice boxes and vignettes are inserted in the book, combined with typical suicide cases, to increase readers' reading interest, help readers understand and grasp the requirements of suicide prevention practice more widely and deeply, and better combine theory and practice.

本书由华中科技大学同济医学院附属协和医院胡德英研究团队主编,得到了医院领导和同事的大力支持,华中科技大学出版社的领导和编辑也为本书付出了辛勤的劳动,在此一并表示衷心感谢!

This book was compiled by the research team with Hu Deying from the Union Hospital of Tongji Medical College of Huazhong University of Science and Technology, under the strong support of the leaders and colleagues of the Union Hospital.

The leaders and editors of Huazhong University of Science and Technology Press have worked hard for this book, and we would like to express sincere thanks.

由于编者能力和水平有限,书中难免存在疏漏和不尽如人意之处。我们真诚希望读者和同道不吝指正,今后将根据意见与建议不断修订完善。

Due to the limited ability of the authors, there will inevitably be omissions and limitations in the book. We sincerely hope that our readers and colleagues will correct us, and we will continue to revise and improve it .